The Scourges of the South? Essays on "The Sickly South" in History, Literature, and Popular Culture

The Scourges of the South? Essays on "The Sickly South" in History, Literature, and Popular Culture

Edited by

Thomas Ærvold Bjerre and Beata Zawadka

CAMBRIDGE SCHOLARS
PUBLISHING

The Scourges of the South?
Essays on "The Sickly South" in History, Literature, and Popular Culture,
Edited by Thomas Ærvold Bjerre and Beata Zawadka

This book first published 2014

Cambridge Scholars Publishing

12 Back Chapman Street, Newcastle upon Tyne, NE6 2XX, UK

British Library Cataloguing in Publication Data
A catalogue record for this book is available from the British Library

ISBN (10): 1-4438-6360-2, ISBN (13): 978-1-4438-6360-5

TABLE OF CONTENTS

Part III: Metaphorical Afflictions

INTRODUCTION

THOMAS ÆRVOLD BJERRE AND BEATA ZAWADKA

"I feel very badly.... I don't know why."
—Katherine Anne Porter, "Pale Horse, Pale Rider"[1]

I

For every admirer of Katherine Anne Porter's oeuvre, the source of the above quotation is not difficult to establish. These words are what the eponymous heroine of Porter's famous *Miranda* series says to an intern from the county hospital arriving to carry her there because of her quickly progressing Spanish flu. Foreshadowed in the story title as the "pale horse, pale rider," the flu—which became a pandemic in 1918 and decimated the world's human resources much like World War I did—first of all stands for a stigma of fatality impressed onto the post-war generation by the experience of mass death. Such a stigma can be interpreted, as it has often been, as a realization that, along with the literally understood mass killings, the existing cultural order and its traditional divides were "exterminated," too, thereby paradoxically offering possibilities of construing a renewed—or ailment-cleansed—system.

In the story this "revitalizing" quality of disease is highlighted in many ways, such as a "war-like" stream of consciousness narration. Through most of the story, Miranda is delirious from high fever, which is mirrored in the slanted, third-person singular narration. This narrative technique, then, might imply her as a "spokesperson" for a system whose chief trait seems to be that it remains "at war" with itself, or else one whose order is perceived as being constantly renewed. Contrived to endlessly re/designing itself, such an "ill" system, once recognized, keeps offering

[1] Katherine Anne Porter, *Pale Horse, Pale Rider: Three Short Novels* (New York: Harcourt Brace & Company 1967), 191. All following quotations from the story "Pale Horse, Pale Rider" are from the same edition of the book.

its participants diverse opportunities for re/inventing themselves in the ways that suit them best, or, as Porter puts it, it gives them "time for everything."[2] However, for the twenty-four-year old Miranda Gay—a southern girl reared to ignore the symptoms suggesting that the "old mortality" of her system might be "unwholesome"—the revelation, via flu, of its diseased constitution is difficult to discern, let alone acknowledge. This learned tunnel vision as regards *status quo* might therefore be a reason why Miranda, even on the way to the hospital, cannot but assess her already critical condition by merely saying, "I feel very badly… I don't know why."[3]

Yet, despite such "critical blindness," Miranda not only manages to live through her illness; by the end of the story she stands ready, it seems, to harness the same blindness in the service of her renewed "healthy" condition. Accordingly, in the parts of the cycle to follow, Miranda resorts to the impaired ("ill") vision of the system she represents so as to come to terms with her past (*The Old Order*) as well as to reorganize the perception of her present ("Holiday"). In this way, by instinctively forging what brought her suffering and pain into an "art of living," Miranda first and foremost demonstrates that even allegedly "ill" heritage can be productively orchestrated and that individual "beneficiaries" of such heritage need not passively accept it as it is. Instead, they can deal with it, be it intuitively, until the moment they feel that the former monolithic construct has been split into many an authorial creation. Since the latter transformation is a harbinger of an "ill" system undergoing democratic changes, it marks the first step towards making a conscious effort at understanding the nature of systemic "illness" and hence at working on maintaining the "culture of health."

The very same idea must have been what guided the EAAS (European Association for American Studies) authorities towards organizing its 2012 biennial conference under the banner of "The Health of the Nation." Held from March 30 to April 2 in Izmir, Turkey, the conference attracted so many scholars from Europe and beyond that it had to be arranged as 24 separate workshops to be further subdivided into panels, a complex structure which immediately suggested the significance of the topic for the contemporary global academic milieu. The variety of the workshop- and panel titles covering the question of health within the American context and referring it to diverse aspects of the American life could not but confirm the significance of the topic in question. Starting from the debates

[2] Ibid., 208.
[3] Ibid., 191.

following the papers read within the frames of the workshop entitled "Physical Hygiene, Mental Health, and the Growth of a Nation: Literature in the Service of Advancing America," to those which cropped up as a result of the discussions on "Hollywood and the Health of the Nation," the notion of health in America was thoroughly examined indeed.[4]

One of the workshops—Workshop 19—entitled "The Scourges of the South" proposed and organized by the Southern Studies Forum of the EAAS discussed the question of health within the context of the American South. For the scholars dealing with the region, the so-called "healthy South" has never been an easy topic. One reason for this might be that, like Miranda in Porter's stories, we have been taught to approach so formulated a topic no further than to the point when it turns out it is a contradiction in terms. On one hand, there is much in the southern history and present situation that indeed justifies such an approach. The region has long been struggling against manifold health issues which still demonstrate as far more serious in the South than in other American regions. Among those issues, physical health problems such as obesity, diabetes and methamphetamine addiction are only the latest to plague the South. Yet, not only that; the South has also been made to bear a lot of metaphorical baggage related to illness. This includes, to name just a few examples, private/public/social/political/cultural/racial/ economic health realized as all types of (un)healthy customs, traditions, manners, morals, rituals, histories and the (un)like southern practices. With all this "misery" in mind, one cannot but consent to Allison Graham's claim that the South continues to function primarily as a "repository of national repressions"[5] and hence a basically "scourge" system.

On the other hand, the same long history of pinpointing the South as a bottomless pit of national ills offers (non)scholars who deal with this field occasions galore to probe into what we have been made to perceive solely as an abyss of America's cultural problems[6] from a host of perspectives. The recent years in particular have seen the appearance of publications on

---

[4] The full list of the workshops and panels organized within the 2012 EAAS conference in Izmir, Turkey can be seen here:
http://www.eaas.eu/images/stories/events/2012/eaas-workshops_izmir-nov_11_2011.pdf

[5] Allison Graham, "The South in Popular Culture," *A Companion to the Literature and Culture of the American South*, eds. Richard Gray and Owen Robinson (Malden, MA: Blackwell Publishing, 2007), 349.

[6] For an extended discussion on the question of the South as America's national problem see e.g. *The South as an American Problem*, eds. Larry J. Griffin and Don H. Doyle (Athens: The University of Georgia Press, 1995).

and of the South which tackle the region's various, allegedly still "ill," aspects as not only an entirely "bad" phenomenon. Rather, a tendency has emerged to posit such "bad" aspects of southern life within what economists today refer to as the space of "endless crisis" and whose consequences they believe are a crucial factor in shaping future generations.[7] Accordingly, the "ill" southern notions such as the prevalence of certain literal and metaphorical, diseases and their "epidemiological patterns;" or natural, literal and metaphorical, "disasters" (e.g. how Katrina/nature/climate but also urbanization, or industrialization have influenced southern "health patterns"); or else the question of mental health in the South including the South's own "midlife crisis," as John Shelton Reed refers to the recent changes in the region,[8] have already received a chance to be "excavated" as not so much problems but the country's cultural opportunities. This, in turn, (re)positions the "scourge" role of the South in American culture in terms of this culture's bountiful gift.

II

This book continues the discussions on the "healthy South" which began in Izmir by exploring the above-mentioned "scourge" role of the region as America's attempt at reinventing her past problems as chances. The discussion on the (un)sickly South is divided into three subsections. Part One ("Bodily Diseases") which interprets illness as a bodily (dis)order comprises essays by Renata Nowaczewska (Szczecin University), Marcel Arbeit (University of Olomouc) and Jan Nordby Gretlund (University of Southern Denmark) respectively. This part of the book opens with Nowaczewska's essay entitled "From 'Gospel of Wealth' to 'Gospel of Health:' The Rockefellers in the South." The selection of this particular article as a sort of a "pilot" for the entire essay collection is not accidental. Analyzing the activity of the Rockefeller Sanitary Commission for the Eradication of Hookworm Disease (1909-1915) that originally worked only in the South, Nowaczewska's paper demonstrates how that activity, designed as a set of preventative measures to be taken against a strictly

---

[7] One fascinating discussion on the subject of the endless crisis is in: Robert Bellamy Foster and Robert W. McChesney, *The Endless Crisis: How Monopoly-Finance Capital Produces Stagnation and Upheaval from USA to China* (Washington: Monthly Review Press, 2012).

[8] See John Shelton Reed, "The South's Midlife Crisis," *Bridging Southern Cultures: An Interdisciplinary Approach*, ed. John Lowe (Baton Rouge: Louisiana State University Press, 2005), p. 254-64.

medical (bodily) problem on a local level soon became an undertaking aimed at improving the knowledge of the pandemic diseases such as hookworm all over the world.

Since that undertaking has been continued till the present day, with other private foundations supporting the program and getting not only state, regional or national authorities but transnational organizations involved as well, it might be considered as explanatory with regard to the knowledge of the entire process of falling "ill." Not only that; the workings of such a process involving means from education to financial aids employed so as to reach the end in question—the "health" of the nation—also metaphorically demarcate the South as a complex, demanding and hence difficult notion having little to do with the region's still commonplace perception as the land of "moonlight and magnolias."

Marcel Arbeit, the author of "Flannery O'Connor's 'The Enduring Chill' as a Medical Tale," the next essay in the collection, seems to confirm that this picture of the American South, with its "defiant" stereotypes, is a persisting discernment of the region. This is visible in Arbeit's decision to interpret the story of the physical and mental health troubles of southern writer Asbury Fox—and of the South that this man represents in the story—as a "medical" rather than a theological case. In this way, Arbeit first and foremost re/reads the "southern situation" in late 1950s American culture as one that, if approached with a healthy dose of rationality, might turn out to be a springboard to the South's hopeful future rather than a continuation of its fate as the national outcast. Thus going against the region's common interpretational grain, Arbeit immediately offers us a way to "heal" its most troublesome "sickness," that is, the general conviction that, in terms of culture interpretation, the South has already been doomed to represent a "lost cause."

The rehabilitative "treatment" of, yet another, southern "lost cause" culture is also the concern of Jan Nordby Gretlund's paper entitled "Years of Discretion: Clyde Edgerton on Old Age;" an essay which closes the first part of this book. The essay tackles the southern idea of old age as Clyde Edgerton, a contemporary writer and native of North Carolina, sees it. According to Gretlund, Edgerton perceives aging in the South primarily as an

> extended period of losses: the loss of memory, the loss of skills, the loss of mobility, the loss of respect, the loss of dignity, the loss of manners, the loss of quality in living, the loss of influence (even on your immediate family), the loss of healthy food, the loss of privacy, the loss of control of your finances, the loss of personal hygiene, the loss of the ability to keep

> clean your much reduced living space, and the loss of the self through the interference of *strangers*."[9]

Added to the questionable gains that old age has in store for the fictional dwellers of Edgertons's South, all these deprivations constitute a fine reason for a culture critic to take a closer look at old age as a "lost cause" indeed.

Gretlund does it by cleverly intertwining in his essay his own analysis of Edgerton's "old age" prose with the actual comments the writer made on it in the course of interviews that he gave to Gretlund in 1996 and 2010. The interviews show that Edgerton's interest in the process of ageing fall back on basically three kinds of stories: those his family told him, those he read, and the ones he observed as a participant in the southern public institution system. Of all these "story sets," none seem to have ever been underwritten by the "happy ending" principle; a blind-eye treatment, as Edgerton himself admits it, only too obviously prompted him to "even up the score"[10] by making old age the leitmotif of his artistic creation, thereby also making ageing a form of art itself. In juxtaposing such an art with the life in the form of making an interview with the presently soon-to-be seventy writer himself a part of a critical analysis of his prose, Gretlund additionally endows this prose—and, with it, the process of ageing—with the power to transcend its "lost cause" status in favor of culturally representing a very "live," or else, "reality-checked" force.

Part Two of this book, titled "Psychological Disorders," deals with the illness understood as mental disturbance, and consists of three essays by Thomas Ærvold Ærvold Bjerre (University of Southern Denmark), Gérald Préher (Université Catholique de Lille), and Susanna Delfino (University of Genoa). The first of these essays entitled "Southern Evil, Southern Violence: Gothic Residues in the Works of William Gay, Barry Hannah, and Cormac McCarthy" by Thomas Ærvold Bjerre introduces the topic of southern madness via an analysis of the Gothic elements in the works of the said southern writers. Bjerre understands these elements collectively as the evil inherent in the region itself that in turn makes itself known to the outside world through the violence of the antagonists. Bjerre further claims that a particular form of this violence, typical for a given

[9] Gretlund, Jan. "Years of Discretion: Clyde Edgerton on Old Age." *The Scourges of the South? Essays on "The Sickly South" in History, Literature, and Popular Culture*, eds. Thomas Ærvold Bjerre and Beata Zawadka (Cambridge: Cambridge Scholars Publishing 2014), 69.

[10] Ibid., 65.

protagonist, corresponds to a particular problem the contemporary southern society suffers from. Yet, not only that; put together, the various types of violence become a collective reason why the South has lost any sense of spirituality.

Starting with the analysis of William Gay's 1999 novel *The Long Home* which introduces to the reader the character of Hardin, the "walkin dead man;"[11] through the analysis of Barry Hannah's 2001 novel *Yonder Stands Your Orphan* featuring the predatory Man Mortimer indicative of a larger southern "zombie culture" of which he is a part; to Cormac McCarthy's well-known novel-made-film *No Country for Old Men* (2005) whose fictional world, permeated by psychopath hitman Anton Chigurh, will "kill you in a heartbeat,"[12] Bjerre leaves the reader no doubt as to what causes the southern mental disturbance: it is the lack of experience that makes one completely "alive," i.e. is meaningful. This (di)spirited state of contemporary "things southern" Bjerre paradoxically ascribes to the increasing role materialism plays in the culture of the region. The fact that he attempts interpreting this culture therefore becomes doubly significant: not only does its interpretation "give body" to what has long been alleged as culturally "incorporeal" but also makes such "(in)corporealness" the very substance of the contemporary southern psychological experience and hence a *sine qua non* of the region's mental (un)disturbance.

One reason why the health of southern mentality has been perceived in so elusive terms might lie in the region's difficulty in (re)inventing its own long gone ideals so that they also embraced the contemporary experience. The practice which, in the words of Louis D. Rubin, can be compared to "get[ting] out from under Faulkner"[13] is the subject of the next essay in the book, Gérald Préher's "Joan Williams and William Faulkner United in Fiction: The Idiot-Connection." The essay analyses a novel and several short stories by Joan Williams, a poet and novelist who was also Faulkner's lover and friend of long standing and whose fiction, Préher claims, has been strongly influenced by Faulkner's oeuvre. Préher takes a particular interest in the influence Faulkner's use of his idiotic characters had on Williams's prose, for he believes that such an influence was a basis for establishing what, throughout his essay, he refers to as the "idiot connection" between the two writers. Since the connection literally rested

---

[11] William Gay, *The Long Home* (Denver, CO.: MacMurray & Beck, 1999), 113.

[12] Cormac McCarthy, *No Country for Old Men* (New York: Alfred A. Knopf, 2005), 271.

[13] Louis D. Rubin, Jr., "The Difficulties of Being a Southern Writer Today: Or, Getting out from under William Faulkner," *The Journal of Southern History* 29, no. 4 (November 1963): 488.

on the fascination the two writers had with characters considered community outcasts, they metaphorically (re)wrote their own illicit and very tormented relationship—and along with it the relationship of the South to the early 20th century America—as a kind of a "world of [its] own," to paraphrase Préher's own phrasing, that is, a space having only so much connection to reality.[14]

Préher demonstrates this by exploring the figure of the loony as it appears first and foremost in Williams's debut novel *The Morning and the Evening* (1961). The loony, Jake, is a retarded mute who is dissociated from the outside world. His muteness makes him unaware of the "difference between the morning and the evening,"[15] as Faulkner himself explained this disability when he considered using the same title that Williams gave her novel for his short story "The Hamlet." As a person with no fixed sense of reality, Jake is therefore an outsider, a position which Préher believes is, on the one hand, an obvious bow Williams took at Faulkner's own loneliness of a writer; *ergo*, he indeed represents the South's own sense of isolation in post-WWI America.

On the other hand, Préher claims that the same isolated perspective filtered through the teller whom Williams, contrary to Faulkner, uses as the story's focalizer rather than narrator makes him and, by extension, the South, a perfect observer of the reality it is a part of. In this way, Jake's—and the southern—"looniness" serves a greater purpose: it also deconstructs the American cultural norms of the time as "loony" because it ostracizes those whose mental patterns did not conform with the mainstream ideals.

Susanna Delfino's essay "Susan P. Grigsby and the Psychological Dimension of Disease and Death in Antebellum and Civil War Kentucky" ends the section on the southern psychological disorders. Here Delfino suggests that the above-mentioned vision of the "loony" South—and the norms which created the vision—have not been limited to the early 20th century. The "loony" image of the region is a creation that extends back to the antebellum period when the South, then a slave region, managed to also come into existence in the national imagination as the "moonlight and magnolias" land. Popularized as a mental pattern, the "loony" double

---

[14] Gérald Préher, "Joan Williams and William Faulkner United in Fiction: The Idiot-Connection," *The Scourges of the South? Essays on "The Sickly South" in History, Literature, and Popular Culture*, eds. Thomas Ærvold Bjerre and Beata Zawadka (Cambridge: Cambridge Scholars Publishing 2014), 102.

[15] Faulkner quoted in Joan Williams, "Faulkner's Advice to a Young Writer," *Faulkner and the Short Story: Faulkner and Yoknapatawpha, 1990*, eds. Evans Harrington and Ann J. Abadie. Jackson (Jackson: University Press of Mississippi, 1992), 256-257.

standard as regards "things southern" that such a split vision of the region entailed, found its realization in many walks of 19th century non/southern life. Delfino analyzes the ground she claims has still remained a veritable *terra incognita* as regards scholarly research: the mental life of white elite southern women.

It has long been highlighted that the everyday life of the woman known as the "plantation mistress" was hardly a bed of magnolia petals. Heavy responsibilities, physical wear, and, added to that, self-sacrifice, culturally expected from women of the planter class at the time in question, are now well-researched and long confirmed reasons for discerning their life as comparable to that of the "slave of the slaves." Yet, few scholars have been occupied with researching the psychological strain that such a life all too obviously generated. Taking as her research material the "virtually untapped" writings of Susan Preston Grigsby, the granddaughter of Kentucky's first governor Isaac Shelby, Delfino explores the devastating effects that the duties of the plantation mistress exerted upon Grigsby's psyche, and how she responded to these tragedies.

Delfino demonstrates that, "repeatedly presented... with major trials such as the death of a child or other kin,"[16] Susan Grigsby never lost control of her emotions even in the most adverse of circumstances such as the Civil War period. Yet, apart from advantages, this indomitable attitude had its price, too. Much as it contributed to her emergence in the postbellum southern reality as an independent woman, invincibility at the same time compelled Susan to disregard her individual sensibility and difficulties, bodily and other, in the name of family survival. This, however, led to her transforming the idea of genteel family respectability and pride into a notion depending on not so much the dynasty-like "illustrious origin" but rather on constantly reworking the meaning of gentility so that it remains tuned up to the outside reality. In so doing, Susan Grigsby—and Susanna Delfino after her—also demonstrated that, when understood as flexibility, the "loony" southern double standard need not be at odds with what we nowadays see and refer to as democratic norms.

In such an egalitarian context, the standard cannot be viewed within the bounds of a mere cultural "norm." Instead it might be read as

---

[16] Susanna Delfino, "Susan P. Grigsby and the Psychological Dimension of Disease and Death in Antebellum and Civil War Kentucky," *The Scourges of the South? Essays on "The Sickly South" in History, Literature, and Popular Culture*, eds. Thomas Ærvold Bjerre and Beata Zawadka (Cambridge: Cambridge Scholars Publishing 2014), 130.

symbolically representing a larger entity—a system, perhaps—whose functioning rests and depends on how it utilizes its *modus operandi*: the "black/white" opposition principle. The third and final part of this book entitled "Metaphorical Affliction" approaches the notion of the southern scourges from precisely this metaphorical angle. This section comprises three essays: "Illness as Metaphor in the American South: Lillian Smith's Diagnosis of a Schizophrenic Culture and a Metastasized Social Body" by Constante González Groba (Universidade de Santiago), "'Don't Turn the Light On!': Tennessee Williams, Illness And Popular Culture" by Richard Hayes (Waterford Institute of Technology), and "The LGBTQ Message in *True Blood* and Charlaine Harris's *Sookie Stackhouse* Novels" by Victoria Amador (American University of Sharjah). In the first of these essays disease as well as the uncleanness which suggestively results from it are discussed as southern political tools used to keep African Americans in line. Groba demonstrates this peculiar segregation practice to have been so pervasive with regard to the southern culture that by the end of the 1950s it eventually mentally underwrote southernness itself as a schizophrenic model.

This model of depriving southerners of an ability to creatively orchestrate the region's cultural energy in a "totalitarian monolith" way rather than as a democratic entity was crying out for some reinvention. Taking as his research material Lillian Smith's writings in which she compares segregation to a cancerous disease (from which she herself suffered for thirteen years), Groba not only metaphorically endorses the "body" of 1950s southern affairs as afflicted or cancerous. He also makes clear, much as Smith did, that in order to be effectively "treated" for such a quickly metastasizing condition as "cancer" (i.e. racism), this "body" must submit to the equally metastasizing, or totalitarian, treatment. Only then can there be a certainty that the system, having been "purged," is ready to be democracy-settled.

Much as such totalitarian systemic treatment resembles infamous cleansing practices (ethnic and other), it also opens possibilities for various cultural groups in the South to voice their own "diseased" conditions. One such "unvoiced" sexuality, which in its repression is "diseased," is the subject of the next essay, Richard Hayes's "Don't Turn the Light On!": Tennessee Williams, Illness and Popular Culture." Hayes interprets the said sexuality as it appears in the selected works of Tennessee Williams and via Susan Sontag's theory of illness as a metaphor that kills. Accordingly, he first and foremost demonstrates how Williams's protagonists' inabilities to manage their own sexual potential in other ways than romantic leads to mental problems represented, in turn, as a sundry of symptoms, from the fear of light to the love of cinema, *ergo*, darkness and the dark forces identified with sexuality.

Following Williams, Hayes pays special attention to the medium of cinema, seeing it as a ubiquitous vehicle that is capable of containing both the "Cinderella myth" and the "adventure of sex." This ubiquity can help transform these apparently incompatible powers so that they would eventually crop up as an entity at once artistic and democratic. In choosing cinema as a way out of the double bind of the sexuality/romanticism loop, Hayes suggests a possible solution to the existing southern tension mentioned above; at the same time he addresses yet another question: that of equality that seems fundamental for the well-being of all cultural groups all over the world and hence for democracy itself, namely, "how to be both alone and companionable at the same time; how to [be] for oneself and an audience and satisfy both; how to treasure the populace and resist populism?"[17]

Victoria Amador's essay entitled "The LGBTQ Message in *True Blood* and Charlaine Harris's *Sookie Stackhouse* Novels," which ends both this part of the book and the entire collection, might be considered as a further clarification of this question. This is because Amador reads the fantasy world of both Harris's novels and HBO's adaptation not so much as a fairy tale but rather an arena where various culturally charged issues are at play. Amador also perceives the popular culture context via which southern cultural politics are filtered as a "safety zone" enabling a discussion of uncomfortable subjects such as racism or homophobia which would otherwise be difficult or simply impossible to undertake. In the last part of her essay, Amador supports this vision of popular culture by providing examples of real life activism that the series and the books spawned. In thus reinventing the fantasy genre and popular culture to which it belongs as worlds with reality effects, and hence, against the grain, Amador also clearly demonstrates that, for the equality to become effective and, consequently, for the world to be "healed" we do not need to eliminate "disease;" we just need to learn to creatively approach it. This collection of essays has been designed as a minute step towards such an understanding of democracy.

---

[17] Richard Hayes, "Don't Turn the Light On!": Tennessee Williams, Illness And Popular Culture," *The Scourges of the South? Essays on "The Sickly South" in History, Literature, and Popular Culture*, eds. Thomas Ærvold Bjerre and Beata Zawadka (Cambridge: Cambridge Scholars Publishing 2014), 161.

Works Cited

"EAAS Workshops, Izmir." http://www.eaas.eu/images/stories/events/2012/eaas-workshops_izmir-nov_11_2011.pdf.

Foster, Robert Bellamy, and Robert W. McChesney. *The Endless Crisis: How Monopoly-Finance Capital Produces Stagnation and Upheaval from USA to China*. Washington: Monthly Review Press 2012.

Graham, Allison. "The South in Popular Culture." *A Companion to the Literature and Culture of the American South*, edited by Richard Gray and Owen Robinson, 335-351. Malden, MA: Blackwell Publishing 2007.

Griffin, Larry J. and Don H. Doyle, eds. *The South as an American Problem*. Athens: The University of Georgia Press 1995.

Porter, Katherine Anne. *Pale Horse, Pale Rider: Three Short Novels*. New York: Harcourt Brace & Company, 1967.

Reed John Shelton. "The South's Midlife Crisis." *Bridging Southern Cultures: An Interdisciplinary Approach*, edited by John Lowe, 254-264. Baton Rouge: Louisiana State University Press, 2005.

Rubin, Jr., Louis D. "The Difficulties of Being a Southern Writer Today: Or, Getting out from under William Faulkner," *The Journal of Southern History* 29, no. 4 (November 1963): 486-494.

Williams, Joan. "Faulkner's Advice to a Young Writer." *Faulkner and the Short Story: Faulkner and Yoknapatawpha, 1990*, edited by Evans Harrington and Ann J. Abadie, 253-262. Jackson: University Press of Mississippi, 1992.

PART I:

BODILY DISEASES

CHAPTER ONE

FROM "GOSPEL OF WEALTH" TO "GOSPEL OF HEALTH": THE ROCKEFELLERS IN THE SOUTH

RENATA NOWACZEWSKA

There are several American private foundations, which have undertaken a variety of programs directed at the inhabitants of the southern states. In the past, their main goal, apart from "the elevation of humankind," was to tackle such issues as education, support of Black colleges, health reform, or eradication of the most troublesome diseases as well as more controversial ones such as eugenics.

The Rockefeller Foundation (RF) has been an unprecedented leader in the field of medical research and medical education. Both the RF and other organizations and research institutes established and generously supported by the Rockefellers have become pathfinders in the improvement of medical training and services provided by doctors or nurses. The RF has pioneered in clinical research, searching for the cure for the niggling, debilitating and the most common illnesses that made entire societies dysfunctional while at the same time increasing and testing this knowledge of preventive measures.

The paper aims at presenting the activities of both the Rockefeller Sanitary Commission for the Eradication of Hookworm Disease (1909-1915), and its successor the International Health Board in the South.

With the help of his main advisor, Frederick Gates, John D. Rockefeller found a simple, workable way of utilizing his amassed fortune for what constituted the promotion of "the well-being of mankind throughout the world,"[1] or "relieving human suffering."[2] He thus exercised

[1] "An Act to Incorporate The Rockefeller Foundation, Charter 488," May 14, 1913, accessed March 22, 2014.

the Gospel of Wealth that had been so successfully preached as a vision of a rich man's obligations by Rockefeller's business competitor Andrew Carnegie. Spiritual in nature, Rockefeller's Gospel was repudiated by the community, media and public opinion. Apparently, Rockefeller's business practices "tainted" the money he offered to benevolent deeds, which resulted in the U.S. government initial refusal to incorporate the RF.[3] In consequence any philanthropic undertaking pursued by the RF should have been as neutral in its scope of interest; as far detached from the Standard Oil Company business endeavors; and as much needed by the society at present and in future as possible.[4] Within such a limited frame of reference, the problem of improving public health appeared to be an acceptable and neutral program. In the opinion of John D. Rockefeller "the best philanthropy involved a search for a cause, an attempt to cure evils at their source."[5] Whereas, the above mentioned F. Gates considered philanthropy as a tool of helping those whose "weaknesses and disabilities erected from causes lying beyond them." Gates demarcated disease as the "supreme ill of human life… and the main source of almost all other human ills, poverty, crime, ignorance, vice, inefficiency, hereditary taint, and many other evils."[6] Thus, the most straightforward way for the Rockefeller

---

http://www.rockefellerfoundation.org/media/download/30ff1883-9e8f-44fd-9dd9-8bf2d6803578, 3.

[2] Rockefeller Archive Center (RAC), Sleepy Hollow, NY, Rockefeller, John D., "Letter from John D. Rockefeller Sr. to Rockefeller Sanitary Commission board members, 1909 October 26," Office of the Messrs. Rockefeller records, series O, Box 52, folder 544. *100 Years: The Rockefeller Foundation*, accessed January 22, 2014, http://rockefeller100.org/items/show/2162.

[3] The US Congress debated the charter for three years and despite many concessions the charter was finally withdrawn. President William Howard Taft disapproved of the establishment of the RF as well. RF charter was incorporated by the NY state legislature with no opposition or criticism. Waldemar A. Nielsen, *The Big Foundations* (New York: Columbia University Press, 1972), 50-52.

[4] The popular charges that JDR's benefactions were planned as a "shield against public censure, … and attempt to reestablish himself and ward off the abuse," according to Raymond Fosdick - an insider of the Rockefeller philanthropic organizations since 1913 and the long-time president of the RF, were not based on facts. He considered it a legend that the Ivy Lee, the public relations counsel, advised JDR to create philanthropic foundations as a "method of establishing himself in public esteem." The firm associated with the Rockefeller philanthropies in 1914, several years after the establishment of the Rockefeller Institute (1901), General Education Board (1903) and the Rockefeller Foundation (1913). Raymond B. Fosdick, *The Story of the Rockefeller Foundation* (New York: Harper, 1952), 4.

[5] Ibid., 22.

[6] Ibid., 23-24.

philanthropies should have led from the Gospel of Wealth to the Gospel of Health: controlling and eliminating communicable diseases to improve public health, first in the U.S. and later on in the entire world.[7]

Gate's views that "science and education [were] the brain and nervous system of civilization, [while] health [was] its heart,"[8] corresponded with those of the modern social reformers. They believed that health conditions were dependent both on the scientific causes of diseases and social problems that lay at the very core of these diseases.[9] The said problems comprised, among others: the lack of proper hygiene often corresponding to poverty, or the lack of knowledge or even ignorance. Therefore, it became clear that prevention and treatment of disease could put an end to poverty and vice. It seemed that the simple way to achieve this was by launching a major campaign educating the public about the causes and effects of certain practices of everyday life and of the lack of adequate hygiene in the households.[10]

Social reformers' belief in high value of public health education stood in opposition to the notion presented and heavily defended by advocates of eugenics who saw no direct advantages coming from such campaigns. They viewed southerners - the addressees of the campaigns as unproductive, solely responsible of the "degeneracy and disease," and as such, hopeless cases as regards any improvement or rehabilitation.[11] The proponents of

---

[7] The Rockefeller Sanitary Commission conducted its work in the South, Latin America, the British Colonies, the Far East and the West Indies, while its successor, the International Health Board initiated its programs in over 80 countries. John Farley, *To Cast Out Disease: A History of the International Health Division of the Rockefeller Foundation, 1913-1951* (Oxford: Oxford University Press, 2004), 4.

[8] Fosdick, *Story*, 23.

[9] "Nineteenth-century hygienists emphasized the social and material environments in which disease developed and advocated both sanitary and social reform as the most effective public health measures." Ann E. Fowler La Berge, *Mission and Method: The Early Nineteenth-Century French Public Health Movement* (Cambridge: Cambridge University Press, 1992), 74.

[10] For more on the concept of disease attributed to the social conditions and the lack of adequate knowledge, see also: Thomas McKeown and C.R. Lowe, *An Introduction to Social Medicine* (Oxford: Blackwell Scientific, 1974), 67-70; Constance A. Nathanson, *Disease Prevention as Social Change The State, Society, and Public Health in the United States, France, Great Britain, and Canada* (New York: Russell Sage Foundation, 2007); Renata Nowaczewska, *Dobroczynna Ameryka* (Warsaw: Warsaw University Press, 2009), Ch. 1.

[11] Matt Wray, *Not Quite White. White Trash and the Boundaries of Whiteness* (Durham and London: Duke University Press, 2006), 101-103. For the discussion

eugenics took their offensive particularly against poor southern whites, who were referred to as "dirt eaters," or "white trash."[12] The prevalent hookworm infection was interpreted as the cause for "the laziness and backwardness" of the southerners. [13]

The New South was supposed to represent a new quality, new values, or a new social standing of the South but most of all an idea capable of attracting the attention of prospective investors from the North.[14] The only thing that stood in the way of the idea being realized was the 2 million of "Crackers," a social group eternally, it seemed, suffering from the hookworm disease.[15] The elites[16] regarded the disease as a myth, even though in some rural areas even 90% of school children were infected.[17] The article in *the New York Times* warned that the wealthy and educated southerners or their families were not immune to the disease, while no progress could be possible without "the enlightened classes carrying along

---

of eugenics practices in the South see: Edward J. Larson, *Sex, Race, and Science: Eugenics in the Deep South* (Baltimore: Johns Hopkins University Press, 1996).

[12] More on the notion of "white trash" or "dirt eating" see: Wray, *Not Quite White*, Introduction and Chapter 4.

[13] Allen Tullos, *Habits of Industry: White Culture and the Transformation of the Carolina Piedmont* (Chapel Hill: UNC Press Books, 1989), 45; John Ettling, *The Germ of Laziness: Rockefeller Philanthropy and Public Health in the New South* (Cambridge: Harvard University Press, 1981), 35-38. The South earned its "reputation for poor health" due to the reoccurring endemic and epidemic outbreaks that earned a well-deserved epithet "scourges of the South." They were caused by various cultural and environmental factors that contributed to southern distinctiveness. Although they were well defined and known to the society and the medical profession, the lack of ability or financial resources thwarted reformers in their attempts to act. James O. Breeden, "Disease as a Factor in Southern Distinctiveness," in *Disease and Distinctiveness in the American South*, ed. Todd L. Savitt, James Harvey Young (Knoxville: The University of Tennessee Press, 1988), 10-13.

[14] The concept of the New South was not only historical, economic or political, but according to M. Wray it was a "set of narratives and myths that southern boosters, politicians, and entrepreneurs invented in order to sell the region to skeptical northern investors." Wray, *Not Quite White,* 171n2.

[15] "Two Million Have Hookworm," *New York Times*, October 13, 1909. The number was of course more of a guess than a correct estimation.

[16] These were not only average well-off southerners but also professionals-doctors, nurses, and health authorities that were so ignorant of the disease and the seriousness of the problem. Fosdick, *Story*, 30.

[17] Robert Shaplen, *Toward the Well-Being of Mankind. Fifty Years of the Rockefeller Foundation* (Garden City, NY: Doubleday & Company, Inc., 1964), 20.

with them the less enlightened and unfortunate classes."[18] In one Virginia school, 38 out of 40 children were infected, while 45 others were too weak to attend school.[19] The earning power of whole families, generation after generation was being reduced by as much as 50% due to the hookworm disease, which made the struggle for existence harder and more hopeless in the South.[20] The general lack of knowledge or awareness of the hazardous for health a condition could also be attributed to the press that commented upon "the lazy germ," "the hookworm theory," "the fad," "the myth" or "the conception of ingenious [Yankee] minds for the injury of the South," or even denounced the assertion that such a disease existed at all.[21] Therefore the challenge lying before doctors, social reformers and public health officials who set out to cope with the disease seemed to be bigger than the disease itself.

The "History" of the Hookworm

The effects of the hookworm disease can be found as early as in ancient times; yet, an Italian physician, Angelo Dubini, discovered the disease itself only in 1838. Between this initial discovery and the year 1843 Dubini conducted several hundred autopsies that helped him identify and name the worm *Ancylostoma duodenale*.[22] Similar observations complemented by descriptions of the possible effects of the hookworm, such as extreme anemia, were made in Egypt and Brazil simultaneously.[23] Since 1878 the hookworm disease was recognized not only at death of a patient during a conducted autopsy but also from ova passed in the feces. The first violent epidemic of anemia happened among men constructing a

---

[18] *New York Times*, October 22, 1909.

[19] Of the 300 examined college students 42% had hookworm. Similar examination conducted in three regiments of state militia revealed 36%, 58% and 32% respectively of infected individuals. Fosdick, *Story*, 30-31.

[20] Shaplen, *Toward the Well-Being,* 24.

[21] RAC, Rockefeller Sanitary Commission for the Eradication of Hookworm Disease records, Wickliffe Rose, "Work of the Rockefeller Sanitary Commission," August 13, 1914, series 1, box 2, folder 33, *100 Years: The Rockefeller Foundation*, accessed January 22, 2014, http://rockefeller100.org/items/show/1874.

[22] Charles Wardell Stiles, *Report upon the Prevalence and Geographic Distribution of Hookworm Disease in the United States* (Washington: Government Printing Office, 1903), 31.

[23] The Rockefeller Foundation, International Health Board, *Bibliography of Hookworm Disease*. Publ. No. 11, (New York: IHB, 1922), xi; Leon Jacobs, "Hookworm Disease." *The American Journal of Nursing* (Nov. 1940): 1191.

tunnel in Italy in 1880. When the malady took place many physicians who went there to examine hundreds of cases pointed to the adverse hygienic conditions as the reasonable cause of the disease.[24]

Not until the discovery of 1.500 worms in the body of a deceased peasant woman in Milan had anyone held parasites to be responsible.[25] In 1913 observations similar to the Italian ones were made among miners in France, Germany, Holland, Belgium, Spain and Hungary. The then infection rate amounted to 13.1% in Germany and to as much as 80% in Spain.[26]

The remedy was hard to find, as the larvae possessed an "enormous resistive power to most known chemical agents."[27] The solution of thymol eventually brought some results allowing the infected patients to be cured after a repeated number of doses were taken. Yet, the process by which people acquired the infection remained unknown until an accidental discovery at Cairo by Professor Arthur Looss. The German scholar, educated in Łódź, Poland, made a serendipity discovery by infecting himself with the hookworm through the skin in 1898.[28] This finding made the control of the hookworm disease very simple. It was enough to avoid direct contact between bare skin, particularly soft places between fingers and toes, and infected mud or water. Thus, the hookworm disease prevention translated into simply avoiding walking barefoot. Prof. Looss published a major monograph on hookworm in 1911 summing up all the knowledge available at that time. He also suggested Thymol and Male Fern as possible, well-known and successful remedies for the disease.[29] In his book he also provided a comprehensive description of the life cycle of the hookworm larvae and its anatomy.

In the New World the first account referring to the new species of hookworm was recorded in 1808. It was Joseph Pitt who in his article discussed dirt eating and anemia cases among "lower class negro and white population" in the American South.[30] Since Pitt's discovery, similar

---

[24] RF, *Bibliography*, xii-xiii.
[25] RF, *The Annual Report of 1917*, 81,
http://www.rockefellerfoundation.org/about-us/annual-reports.
[26] RF, *Bibliography,* xv-xvii; RF, *Annual Report 1917*, 147-149.
[27] RF, *Bibliography*, xiv.
[28] "The Death of Arthur Looss," *American Journal of Public Health,* 13, no. 8 (August 1923): 659-659.
[29] RF, *Bibliography*, vii, xviii.
[30] Joseph Pitt, "Observations on the Country and Diseases near Roanoke River, in the State of North-Carolina," *New York Medical Repository* 5 (1808): 340-1, quoted in: RF, *Bibliography*, xix

cases were reported and discussed in scientific literature until 1902 when Dr. Charles Wardell Stiles named the new species *Necator Americanus*, meaning "the American killer." Also known as "the American hookworm," the parasite was most probably carried to America from Africa by slaves.[31] The first investigation of the massive cases of anemia was conducted in Puerto Rico in 1904. [32]

The symptoms of being infected with the American hookworm included itching ("ground itch" or "dew itch") as larvae penetrated through the pulmonary tract, and severe anemia caused by the destruction of red blood cells by the adult worm attached to intestinal mucosa and because of the toxic substances introduced into the body either directly or indirectly by the parasite.[33] Generally, the appetite was increased, and there was a desire for bulky foods, which might have got perverted into a craving for eating earth and all sorts of unnatural things, such as paper, slate pencils, coffee grounds and ashes. Dirt eating was quite a common symptom of the hookworm disease and "pot bellies" resulting from this habit could often be seen in severe hookworm cases.[34] Other symptoms included dry and pale skin, palpitation, irritation of the larynx, headache, tiredness and exhaustion (confused with laziness).[35] "Eyes [were] without color or sparkle and expressions stupid and intensely melancholy," sex organs of the infected children were underdeveloped, mental growth hindered, males lost sexual power while females had irregular menstruation.[36]

Also, dullness in school and a lack of desire to continue one's education were common among hookworm-infected children. In adults the mental attitude was one of apathy and melancholy, stupidity and lack of concentrative ability. Shiftlessness, laziness, lack of ability to understand and to improve themselves were the effects which were at least in part produced by the hookworm on people who would otherwise be progressive

---

[31] RF, *Bibliography,* xix; Jacobs, "Hookworm Disease," 1191.

[32] RF, *Bibliography, xx.*

[33] Mary Boccacio,"Ground Itch and Dew Poison: The Rockefeller Sanitary Commission, 1909-1914," *Journal of Medicine and Allied Sciences*, 27, no. 1 (1972): 31; Florence O. Gibbs, "Uncinariasis or Hookworm Disease," *The American Journal of Nursing*, 13, no. 6 (March 1913): 439; Tood L. Savitt, *Medicine and Slavery. The Diseases and Health Care of Blacks in Antebellum Virginia* (Urbana: University of Illinois Press, 1978), 70.

[34] Ettling, *Germ of Laziness*, 35.

[35] Martha M. Giltner, "Hookworm Disease: A Health Problem of the South," *The American Journal of Nursing*, 22, no. 10 (July 1922): 806-7; Jacobs, "Hookworm Disease," 1193.

[36] Savitt, *Medicine and Slavery*, 69-71; Gibbs, "Uncinariasis or Hookworm Disease," 440.

and strong. Going barefoot on land that had been contaminated with human feces was one of the main ways of acquiring the parasite.[37] The manner in which feces were disposed of in the South, meaning no or few box privies that were not properly taken care of, was the main reason why more infections were observed in rural areas. [38]

A person once diagnosed could require treatment up to four times, so in many cases a patient would be given medicine in precise doses ascribed to his/her age together with the instructions how to use it at home.[39] As the treatment was a true nuisance, unpleasant and at times even painful (for it involved refraining from consuming alcohol, fat or oil, including milk and alcohol-containing medicine so as to avoid thymol poisoning, and was followed by frequent intestine evacuation with the help of Epsom salts) the treatment was advised to be conducted on Saturdays and Sundays as an average patient "could not afford losing several days' wages."[40]

The Hookworm Campaign

The problem of the hookworm disease in the South was brought to the attention of the Rockefellers by an incident when President of the General Education Board[41] Dr. Wallace Buttrick met Dr. Charles Wardell Stiles, who "put up the biggest proposition ever to the Rockefeller office."[42] The need to eradicate the debilitating disease and to set up new standards for

[37] Jacobs, "Hookworm Disease," 1191-6.

[38] Stiles, *Report upon Hookworm Disease*, 50.

[39] Charles Wardell Stiles and George F. Leonard "Administration of Thymol in Hookworm Disease," *Public Health Reports* (1896-1970), 26, no. 49 (Dec. 8, 1911): 1925.

[40] Stiles, *Report upon Hookworm Disease*, 86-89; Ch. W. Stiles, "The Treatment of Hookworm Disease," *Public Health Reports* (1896-1970) 24, no. 34 (Aug. 20, 1909): 1191-1193.

[41] Both JDR and his son John, Jr. had been interested in the "Negro problem" for a long time. The latter since his teens as his mother's parents, Harvey Buel Spelman and Lucy Henry Spelman were actively involved in the Underground Railroad, while his mother, JDR's wife, was an abolitionist herself. All Rockefellers pursued the aim of improving education for the Southern Blacks. For the purpose of improving educational system, with special emphasis on the South and the education of Blacks, the General Education Board was established in 1903. The Rockefellers also supported the Spelman College that was renamed in honor of Laura Spelman, JDR's wife. Fosdick, *Story*, 9. For more on the General Education Board, see:
http://rockefeller100.org/exhibits/show/education/general_education_board.

[42] Fosdick, *Story*, 10.

the public health led to the establishment of the Rockefeller Sanitary Commission in 1909.[43] It was only the "dramatic success" of the RSC in eliminating the hookworm disease in the South that made the RF establish International Health Board and extend the hookworm campaign to other parts of the world, in order to create "agencies for the promotion of public sanitation and the spread of the knowledge of scientific medicine."[44] Beginning with the West Indies and Latin America this program was eventually extended to 53 countries and 29 islands.[45] In 1916 the Board was expanded and renamed International Health Division, which eventually became "the world's most important agent of public health work before WHO was created."[46]

Since the very beginning the Rockefeller Foundation seemed to be doomed to success. It got engaged in the programs combating the most common, but curable perils of contemporary society that till then had been left at the verge of any institution's, society's or authorities' interest.[47]

---

[43] Except the campaign to eradicate the hookworm disease, the RSC was interested in organizing a well-funded public health network across the USA. In the South, where the issue was particularly neglected, there were only 3 state departments of health and very few full-time health officers. RAC, Rockefeller Foundation, Excerpt from Trustees Bulletin, "Development of Rural Health Services," December 1939, RG 3, Series 908, Box 14, File 149. *100 Years: The Rockefeller Foundation*, accessed January 21, 2014, http://rockefeller100.org/items/show/2172.

[44] RAC, The Rockefeller Foundation, "Resolutions Establishing the International Health Commission," June 27, 1913. Administration, Program and Policy, RG 3.1, series 900, box 18, folder 129. *100 Years: The Rockefeller Foundation*, accessed January 22, 2014, http://rockefeller100.org/items/show/2159.

[45] Jules Abels, *The Rockefeller Billions: The Story of the World's Most Stupendous Fortune* (New York: Macmillan, 1965), 330. The RF supported local health authorities in anti-hookworm programs in the US and in many foreign countries providing required financial resources and supervising the campaigns. RF, *Annual Report 1929*, 101. IHC operated in Latin America in countries as: Brazil, Mauritius, Colombia; in Europe: Spain, France, Holland, Germany, Belgium, Hungary, Italy, mostly in the mining districts. RF, *The Annual Report of 1917*, 150; *The Annual Report of 1918*, 35; *The Annual of Report 1920*, 139, 141, 143, 379; all available at: http://www.rockefellerfoundation.org/about-us/annual-reports.

[46] John Farley, *To Cast Out Disease*, 2. On the RF workings for the eradication of the hookworm disease (part 1), yellow fever, and malaria see: William Greer, *The Plague Killers* (New York: Scribner's, 1969).

[47] Several of the organizations and institutions, under the auspices of the RF or the mentioned GEB, were established for the purpose of improving general knowledge on causes, cure and prevention of common diseases, through public health reform,

These perils ranged from the debilitating hookworm disease, through deadly malaria, to industrial relations and problems of the ageing American society and the much-needed security at the old age.[48] The proposed campaign to eradicate hookworm disease was demanding due to a lack of any national programs, international standards or even public resources to fund, examine, and collect data on major public health threats and to conduct control, prevention and education programs.[49] The Rockefeller Foundation was the first to undertake the large-scope programs of health prevention and public health education.

Dr. Charles Stiles, a U.S. Public Health Service physician, had been trying for a long time to draw some attention to the role hookworm was playing in widespread lethargy among cotton mill workers in the southern states. While in the antebellum South hookworm was "mostly limited to slaves and a very small class of poor whites, the postwar poverty exposed growing number of southerners to hookworm infection, making it a major threat to regional health."[50] Thus, when John D. Rockefeller asked several most noted medical specialists if there was a disease affecting large

---

medical research, public health education and training. The long list of sponsored programs and institutions includes: Rockefeller Institute for Medical Research, Johns Hopkins University School of Medicine, American Medical Association, The American Social Hygiene Association, National Committee for the Improvement of Nursing Services. The RF also helped improve medical and nursing education abroad, in China- Peking Union Medical College, in India- All India School of Hygiene and Public Health, and similar schools in Europe and other parts of the world: Zagreb, Lyon, Budapest, Warsaw, Tokyo, London, San Paolo. Compare: RF, *The Annual Reports* available at: http://www.rockefellerfoundation.org/about-us/annual-reports or the Rockefeller Foundation centennial at: http://rockefeller100.org/.

[48] On the RF's role in labor relations, social security act or the creation and financing of the Social Science Research Council, the Industrial Relations Section and the Industrial Relation Counselors, see: G. William Domhoff, *State Autonomy or Class Dominance? Case Studies on Policy Making in America* (New York: Aldine Transaction, 1996), Ch. 5, 117-149.

[49] The first health reform at the state level was initiated by the Progressives, though no national health programs were implemented until the first social welfare acts during the New Deal had been passed. Beatrix Hoffman, "Health Care Reform and Social Movements in the United States." *American Journal of Public Health.* 93(1), (Jan., 2003): 75–85. On the lack of the federally sponsored programs, see: Alan Derickson, *Health Security for All: Dreams of Universal Health Care in America* (Baltimore: Johns Hopkins University Press, 2005), Ch. 3.

[50] James O. Breeden, "Science and Medicine," in *Encyclopedia of Southern Culture*, ed. Charles R. Wilson and William Ferris (Chapel Hill: University of N.C. Press, 1989), 1340-41.

numbers of people of which they could say "I know all about this and I can cure it, not in fifty or even eighty percent of the cases, but in one hundred percent,"[51] Stiles' efforts with "pinpointing" the hookworm problem could come to his aid. The campaign's success would have guaranteed far-reaching results,[52] although it brought much suspicion that the Rockefellers initiated the whole campaign because they wanted to go into the shoe business,[53] producing shoes for the barefooted Southern whites to protect them from infections while walking on the polluted soil.

The gift of $1 million by John D. Rockefeller to eradicate hookworm disease was announced on October 26, 1909. The commission to administer the gift consisted of Rockefeller's closest advisors, scientists and social reformers.[54] The Rockefeller Commission for the Eradication of Hookworm Disease (RSC) was called into action only after "the cure and prevention" had been effectively demonstrated as bringing positive results.[55] The commission members exhibited a progressive view that could draw the attention of investors in the South. The commission attempted to convince industrialists that the disease itself could retard the physical and mental development of the infected workers making their

---

[51] Peter Collier and David Horowitz, *The Rockefellers: An American Dynasty* (New York: Holt, Rinehart and Winston, 1976).

[52] Victor Heiser, *An American Doctor's Odyssey* (New York: W. W. Norton & Co Inc., 1936), 268.

[53] Shaplen, *Toward the Well-Being*, 21.

[54]. Dr. William H. Welch, Professor of Pathology in Johns Hopkins University and President of the American Medical Association; Dr. Simon Flexner, Director of Rockefeller Institute for Medical Research; the mentioned Dr. Ch. Wardell Stiles, Chief of the Division of Zoology, United States Public Health and Marine Hospital Service, discoverer of the prevalence of the disease in America; Dr. Edwin A. Alderman, President of the University of Virginia; Dr. David F. Houston, Chancellor of Washington University, St. Louis, Mo; Professor P. P. Claxton, Professor of Education in the University of Tennessee; J. Y. Joyner, State Superintendent of Education in North Carolina and President of the National Educational Association; Walter H. Page, Editor of the *World's Work*; Dr. H. B. Frissell, Principal of the Hampton Institute; Frederick T. Gates, one of Rockefeller's business managers; Starr J. Murphy, Rockefeller's Counsel in benevolent matters and his son John D. Rockefeller, Jr. "Rockefeller Gift to Kill 'Hookworm': Million-Dollar Fund to be Spent by a Commission." *New York Times* (October 29, 1909): 1.

[55] RAC, John D. Rockefeller, "Letter from John D. Rockefeller Sr. to Rockefeller Sanitary Commission board members, 1909 October 26," Office of the Messrs. Rockefeller records, series O, box 52, folder 544. *100 Years: The Rockefeller Foundation*, accessed January 25, 2014,
http://rockefeller100.org/items/show/2163, 1.

labor less efficient.[56] Added to the death toll from pneumonia, typhoid fever and malaria, the hookworm disease was another factor seriously jeopardizing the economic development of the region, an argument which was frequently repeated and so not quite strange to Rockefeller's stance towards labor force. Furthermore, the Commission stressed that the disease, though hitting the school children the hardest, left few safe. With an estimated 2 million of southerners infected, the disease posed a danger to all classes and races.[57] However, in RSC reports there are frequent references to the strange approach of southerners who firmly insisted that the Commission workers would limit the examination and treatment to poor whites only, quoting studies indicating that blacks were "much less susceptible to hookworm disease, cystic fibrosis, and skin cancer than Caucasians."[58]

The selection process of the states to which the campaign should be directed was not straightforward. First, the RSC searched the existing state records for the health reports in respect to the highest degree of possible hookworm cases. The search eventuated in the selection of 11 Southern states (Alabama, Arkansas, Georgia, Kentucky, Louisiana, Mississippi, North Carolina, South Carolina, Tennessee, Texas and Virginia) out of which 9 with the highest level of infections, reaching as much as 90% of infected population in some counties, were picked. The states in question were the following: Virginia, North and South Carolina, Georgia, Tennessee, Arkansas, Mississippi, Alabama and Louisiana.[59] The Commission's activities, mostly lectures, exhibits and demonstrations convincing the public and health officials about the urgent need to

---

[56] On the "profitability" of healthy workers as employer's "human capital, see: Richard E. Brown, *Rockefeller Medicine Men: Medicine and Capitalism in America* (Berkley: University of California Press, 1979), Ch. 3.

[57] RAC, Rockefeller Sanitary Commission for the Eradication of Hookworm Disease, "Letter from Rockefeller Sanitary Commission board members to John D. Rockefeller Sr., 1909 October 26," Office of the Messrs. Rockefeller records, series O, box 52, folder 544, *100 Years: The Rockefeller Foundation*, accessed January 25, 2014, http://rockefeller100.org/items/show/2162; "Commission's Reply to John D. Rockefeller," (AAAS), *Science* 30, no. 775 (Nov. 5, 1909): 636.

[58] Todd L. Savitt, *Medicine and Slavery. The Diseases and Health Care of Blacks in Antebellum Virginia* (Urbana: University of Illinois Press, 1978), 46. Dr. Stiles also noticed fewer cases of blacks getting infected but could not point to the plausible cause of that except that houses of black families were cleaner and that children were given "worm tea" to expel the "eelworm or calomel to regulate the liver." Stiles, *Report upon Hookworm Disease*, 52.

[59] By 1914, Texas and Kentucky established their own programs and surveys.

eradicate the hookworm disease, were based on the philosophy that the Rockefeller organization should be "a partner, but not a patron," working through governments in 653 out of 1,142 counties.[60]

The mentioned compilation of reports and records for the RSC was a highly frustrating task to perform. Wickliffe Rose, the executive secretary of the RSC,[61] complained that the performance of this task "lacked uniformity in the maintenance of records made," a fact, which almost disabled the providing of the actual numbers of people that were examined and later, treated. Having a million dollar budget to spend, Rose strived to dispose of it undertaking the biggest administrative and medical challenge of aiding 2 million infected southerners. In spite both of the great suspicion and hostility on the part of businessmen and the ignorance of the masses, the southern public health movement managed to push the reforms to a broad front.[62]

Apart from monetary contributions from the local governments, the "aggressive campaign"[63] to eradicate hookworm required expert and technical support of medical schools, nursing and training staff, social workers and many more. It could not have been successful without substantial and quite often voluntary help provided by public officials, public school teachers, doctor's associations, school boards, and all the forces that the RSC managed to activate. The campaign got many willing contributors and participants involved. Newspapers posted announcements of free examinations taking place in mobile dispensaries; ministers encouraged congregation members just as employers encouraged their workers to participate.[64] Women's clubs in the South exhorted the biggest support, while schools were subjected to mandatory examinations.[65] Southern rural communities were instructed in the consequences of the

---

[60] RF, *The Annual Report of 1916*, 89-90.

[61] After the hookworm campaign was commenced in 1915 Rose was nominated to become the Director of the International Health Board, the post he held until 1923. Rose had worked for Peabody and Slater Funds before coming to RSC. A southerner himself, he became one of the first professional (and extremely meticulous) bureaucrats devoted to the mission of bringing change in the South. RAC, "Wickliffe Rose," accessed March 22, 2014, http://rockefeller100.org/biography/show/wickliffe-rose; The Tennessee Encyclopedia of History and Culture, "Wickliff Rose," accessed March 22, 2014, http://tennesseeencyclopedia.net/entry.php?rec=1150.

[62] Breeden, "Science and Medicine," 1341.

[63] "To Study the Hookworm," *Chicago Daily Tribune* Oct 30, 1909, 10.

[64] RF, *The Annual Report of 1916*, 77-80.

[65] For more on the cooperation of women's clubs, farmers' unions and insurance companies, see: Boccaccio, "Ground Itch and Dew Poison," 38-40.

hookworm infection, the parasites' cycles but most of all of the desired hygienic practices and habits. The RF used a special exhibit material to illustrate the story of the hookworm disease to be used by public health boards. The material included a durable lecture charts for schools, a collection of fifty lantern slides, photos, specimen of hookworm to be presented and leaflets, letters, pamphlets, notices, and bulletins.[66] Demonstrations drew much attention; enthusiasm and activity to remote areas, while initial embarrassment was gone once the examined individuals had discovered how many people were infected.[67]

Rockefeller workers were using all possible means to reach the public, addressing people at county fairs, and inviting folks to "Come Out, Bring Your Family, Spend the Day, and Hear the Doctor Talk."[68] However, of these means, the microscope turned out to be the best educational instrument displaying to the skeptic the eggs or the larvae of the hookworm. In the campaign, the public learned the simple hookworm prevention methods such as wearing shoes, not walking on polluted ground, avoiding dirty water reservoirs, and building proper privies.

In the survey conducted in 770 southern counties between 1912-1915 (when the RSC program had already been under way for at least three years) it was discovered that only 0.6% of inspected 287,606 farm houses had "satisfactory provisions for the prevention of soil contamination," i.e., sanitary privies, while almost half had none at all. The sanitary conditions in public buildings were equally appalling, for they most often had one privy or none at all at people's disposal. For example, in South Carolina only 0.4% of houses had a sanitary outhouse, while Tennessee had as few as 0.3%.[69]

The survey eventually developed into a study on the efficiency of various types of latrines, conducted under the Rockefeller Institutes for Medical Research. The institute provided a sketch of a sanitary privy to be built in rural areas of the South so as to prevent typhoid, dysentery, diarrhea and other enteric infections from spreading as the result of a widespread custom of polluting the soil with human feces.[70] Of the 20,515 homes inspected between 1914 and 1916, 555 homes were provided with the appropriate type of latrine at the first inspection, 12,337 at the last

[66] RF, *The Annual Report of 1916*, 57-8, 98-9. The total of literature distributed in a single year of 1916 reached 54,334 pieces. The total number of lectures given amounted to 705 in which 43,623 people participated.
[67] Boccaccio, "Ground Itch and Dew Poison," 43.
[68] Shaplen, *Toward the Well-Being*, 22.
[69] RF, *The Annual Report of 1917*, 138; Shaplen, *Toward the Well-Being*, 29.
[70] RF, *The Annual Report of 1916*, 64, 78.

inspection and 4,939 built new latrines.[71] Inhabitants of South Carolina and Mississippi built the biggest numbers of outhouses, probably due to a new practice of publishing the names of families who had the proper standard latrines. A map giving the location of all such houses followed it. The list included the names of both whites and colored.[72]

A highly effective way of addressing the public was via the use of the educational drama created by the International Health Board in 1920 entitled "Unhooking the Hookworm." This short movie is an educational presentation of the disease as experienced by a white Southern family. The movie starts with a scene in which a boy, pale looking and very apathetic, is lying on the porch of his house. He is weak and "too tired" to play with his friend. The film pauses several times explaining that the reason for this boy's strange behavior; i.e., that he is lethargic is the hookworm infection. The movie subsequently gives a detailed explanation of the possible ways humans can get infected with the hookworm; of the way the worm enters and leaves the body; of the damages it causes to organs, and of the symptoms and methods of curing the disease. After the boy's father takes him to the doctor to be treated, the boy recovers to full health and the movie ends with an optimistic scene of him joining his friends swimming in a river.[73] Previous proposed versions of the movie were less idyllic and suggested violence and criminal activity within the family. Many reviewers were of the opinion that the movie should focus on workers and not the rural communities, presenting the loss of manpower due to the disease.[74] Others pointed to other educational resources presented by the RSC; the movie presented only white rural inhabitants and totally ignoring the black population. The movie did not appeal to black people; on the contrary; seeing "a partially exposed white person" they got distracted and burst into laughter. [75]

---

[71] Ibid., 94-5.

[72] Ibid., 85; "Forrest County Leads the State in Rural Sanitation," *The Tribune*, Hattiesburg, Miss. July 23, 1916, quoted in RF, *The Annual Report of 1916*, 83.

[73] The movie available at: RAC, "Unhooking the Hookworm," accessed March 22, 2014, http://www.rockarch.org/feature/hookworm.php.

[74] RAC, Rockefeller Foundation, "Preliminary Draft of Plan for Production of a Film on Hookworm Disease" Sept 12, 1917, RG 1.1, Series 100: International, 1913-1958, Box 5, Folder 42, *Films-Reports 1917-1927*, part 3; RAC, Rockefeller Foundation, "Tentative Scenario for Moving-Picture Film No. 2," RG 5, Series 1.2, Box 20, Folder 302, *938 – Films – General and Individual, 1914*.

[75] RAC, Rockefeller Foundation, "A Letter to John Ferrell," December 17, 1923, IHB/ Division records, RG 5, Subseries 1.01: Correspondence, General 1910-1927, Box 69, Folder 971.

On launching the hookworm eradication campaign in other parts of the world by the IHB, the film was translated into Spanish, French and Portuguese and distributed in many Asian countries, Latin America, Australia and Oceania.[76] The Rockefeller Foundation adhering to a belief that "progress is dependent primarily on trained men who are natives of the country in which the public health measures are to be affected," decided to increase funds for rural health work, health services, and education initiatives, once the direct operation costs of the hookworm campaign started decreasing.[77]

The biggest success noted by the RF was an increase in the state health funds. Between 1910 and 1915 they rose by 136%, with North Carolina's funds increasing from $12,500 to $150,000 and South Carolina's from $24,000 to $75,000.[78] The general appropriations to the State Boards of Health grew from $255,395 in 1910 to $1,416,111 in 1918. The effect was that a number of new infections in 35 counties got lowered by 11%, thus the number of infected persons was reduced by approximately one-third.[79]

Evaluating the campaign it must be stressed that, unfortunately, too much pressure was put on the achievement of the results. It seems that the public health officers were calculating the number of examined individuals rather than full recovery cases. This pressure distorted the image of the campaign as representative of a major competition between doctors, each struggling to treat the biggest possible number of patients.[80] In consequence, many people who needed a repeated treatment would only be given medicine. There was no guarantee, however, they would take it or the treatment would be fully successful. Similarly, there was no assurance that when the campaign was announced to be finished, the purpose of curing the South had been fulfilled. The RSC was chartered for five years, and when it was time to complete the program, Wickliffe Rose was keen on extending it, for he knew how much work remained undone. It was acknowledged that the medical profession and the general public recognized "the prevalence of hookworm disease and regard its cure and

---

[76] RAC, "Unhooking the Hookworm."

[77] "The Rockefeller Report," *New York Times* Nov. 12, 1929, 29.

[78] Since 1916, the state and county authorities provided 50-75% of funds for the procedures of eradicating the hookworm while the remaining amount came from IHB. RF, *The Annual Report of 1916*, 88-9.

[79] RF, *The Annual Report of 1916*, 89, 93-99; RF, *The Annual Report of 1917*, 169.

[80] Boccaccio, "Ground Itch and Dew Poison," 52. It is difficult to evaluate the partnership between the RSC and the state boards of health due to the lack of "uniform record keeping," because some officers would "lump some figures together, give others in detail, and ignore still other completely." Ibid.

prevention as an essential part of public health work in the South."[81] "Interest had been awakened, state machinery built up, and the program, by and large, accomplished."[82] The Commission's aim was demonstration only, and when "reasonable local enlightenment has created the local responsibility for self help,"[83] that was an achievement and a sign to move on and extend the work elsewhere.

There might be several possible reasons for the hookworm eradication campaign to take place in the South. Firstly, the expanding industry "promising progress and prosperity based on the northern model,"[84] needed healthy, highly productive and willing workers who would be able to perform their tasks and responsibilities effectively.[85] Similarly, the U.S. army rejected recruits from the South because they harbored pests and were even too weak to survive through the initial training. Also, a tropical disease that originated in Africa was more successful in bringing national attention to the South as a "sick, sinful" and forgotten section of the US. However, according to many a critic the campaign was not public health philanthropy but a "secularized missionary work" becoming a springboard for the global activities of Rockefeller do-gooders.[86]

Of course, the emerging bourgeois society of the Piedmont in the 1880s-1900s was equally influential a force in implementing national public health or education standards. Merchants, lawyers, editors, doctors and bankers were getting increasingly involved in the region's affairs and programs such as compulsory inoculations or free white public schooling. Such campaigns were not only for the betterment of the poor whites or blacks, disfranchised, economically discriminated but also they reflected attitudes of the new southerners backed up by enterprising northerners seeking new undertakings in the South.[87] The improvements were directed

---

[81] Dr. W. Rose, administration secretary of the RSC quoted in Fosdick, *Story*, 10.

[82] F.T. Gates to J.D. Rockefeller, 19 August 1914, RF, quoted in Boccaccio, "Ground Itch and Dew Poison," 51.

[83] F.T. Gates to W. Rose, 21 August 1914, RSC, quoted in Boccaccio, "Ground Itch and Dew Poison," 51.

[84] Breeden, "Science and Medicine," 1340.

[85] On improved efficiency of cured workers in the South and "economic importance of the hookworm disease," see: Boccaccio, "Ground Itch and Dew Poison," 40 and Stiles, *Report upon Hookworm Disease*, 96-97.

[86] Allen Tullos, "The Germ of Laziness: Rockefeller Philanthropy and Public Health in the New South, by John Ettling, Harvard University Press, 1981. A Review," *The Journal of the Southern Regional Council*, 1978-2003 4, no. 6 (1982): 15-17.

[87] Ibid., 16-17.

by the *laissez faire* approach, new managerial practices, and the concept of keeping certain benefits to the right classes.

Rockefeller's gift seemed to correspond with this line of thinking for it was a malady eradication project directed to the Southern states specifically, not because they were hit the hardest but because "John D. Rockefeller had had a pleasure of spending a portion of each year" in the region, doing business and resting. It was a sign of his "appreciation of the many kindnesses and hospitalities" shown by the southerners.[88]

With all the shortcomings of the RSC record compilation and keeping, it was the first public health record system in the U.S. kept on such a large scale. It resulted in the development of a regular reporting system via which health departments on state and local levels provided, among others, weekly figures of new occurrences of diseases and the conditions under which they spread.[89] This, in turn, helped reduce the number of infections and increased the general knowledge of hygiene and health habits in the South. After the system had been developed in the States, the RF could move on to more challenging tasks and overseas territories such as the colonial possessions of Great Britain,[90] drawing the attention of a wider, international audience to the generosity of the Rockefeller wealth.

Works Cited

"An Act to Incorporate The Rockefeller Foundation, Charter 488," May 14, 1913. Accessed March 22, 2014. http://www.rockefellerfoundation.org/media/download/30ff1883-9e8f-44fd-9dd9-8bf2d6803578.

Abels, Jules. *The Rockefeller Billions: The Story of the World's Most Stupendous Fortune*. New York: Macmillan, 1965.

---

88 RAC, J.D. Rockefeller, "Letter from John D. Rockefeller Sr. to Rockefeller Sanitary Commission," 2.

89 The Public Health Reports published weekly summaries of cases reported by states that provided the exact number of cases, number of deaths caused by communicable diseases and the distribution of cases by states and cities. Compare "Health Prevalence of Disease," reports for the week ended October 30, 1920 and November 6, 1920: 2722-2748.

90 In one of the regions the infection rate amounted to 52%-75% of general population, depending on the district; 70%-90% for plantation laborers and 65%-90% for Indian immigrants to the colonies. Shirish N. Kavadi, "'Parasites Lost and Parasites Regained' Rockefeller Foundation's Anti-Hookworm Campaign in Madras Presidency," *Economic & Political Weekly*, 42(2), (Jan. 13, 2007): 130-137.

Boccacio, Mary. "Ground Itch and Dew Poison: The Rockefeller Sanitary Commission, 1909-1914," *Journal of Medicine and Allied Sciences* 27, no. 1 (1972): 30-53.

Breeden, James O. "Disease as a Factor in Southern Distinctiveness." *Disease and Distinctiveness in the American South,* edited by. Todd L. Savitt and James Harvey Young, 1-28. Knoxville: The University of Tennessee Press, 1988.

—. "Science and Medicine." *Encyclopedia of Southern Culture*, edited by Charles R. Wilson and William Ferris, 1340-41. Chapel Hill: University of North Carolina Press, 1989.

Brown, E. Richard. *Rockefeller Medicine Men: Medicine and Capitalism in America*. Berkley: University of California Press, 1979.

Collier, Peter and David Horowitz. *The Rockefellers: An American Dynasty*. New York: Holt, Rinehart and Winston, 1976.

"Commission's Reply to John D. Rockefeller," (AAAS), *Science* 30, no. 775 (Nov. 5, 1909): 636.

Derickson, Alan. *Health Security for All: Dreams of Universal Health Care in America.* Baltimore: Johns Hopkins University Press, 2005.

Domhoff, G. William. *State Autonomy or Class Dominance? Case Studies on Policy Making in America*. New York: Aldine Transaction, 1996.

"The Death of Arthur Looss." *American Journal of Public Health* 13, no. 8 (August 1923): 659-659.

Ettling, John. *The Germ of Laziness: Rockefeller Philanthropy and Public Health in the New South.* Cambridge: Harvard University Press, 1981.

Farley, John. *To Cast Out Disease: A History of the International Health Division of the Rockefeller Foundation, 1913-1951*. Oxford: Oxford University Press, 2004.

Fosdick, Raymond B. *The Story of the Rockefeller Foundation*. New York: Harper, 1952.

"Forrest County Leads the State in Rural Sanitation," *The Tribune*, Hattiesburg, Miss. July 23, 1916.

Gibbs, Florence O. "Uncinariasis or Hookworm Disease," *The American Journal of Nursing* 13, no. 6 (March 1913): 438-442.

Giltner, Martha, M. "Hookworm Disease: A Health Problem of the South." *The American Journal of Nursing* 22, no. 10 (July 1922): 804-7.

Greer, William. *The Plague Killers.* New York: Scribner's, 1969.

Heiser, Victor. *An American Doctor's Odyssey: Adventures in Forty-Five Countries*. New York: W. W. Norton & Co Inc., 1936.

"Health Prevalence of Disease: United States." *Public Health Reports* (1896-1970), 35(46), (Nov. 12, 1920): 2722-2748.

Hoffman, Beatrix. "Health Care Reform and Social Movements in the United States." *American Journal of Public Health* 93, no. 1 (2003 January): 75–85

Jacobs, Leon. "Hookworm Disease." *The American Journal of Nursing* 40, no. 11 (Nov. 1940): 1191-1196.

Kavadi, Shirish N. "'Parasites Lost and Parasites Regained' Rockefeller Foundation's Anti-Hookworm Campaign in Madras Presidency." *Economic & Political Weekly*, 42(2), (Jan. 13, 2007): 130-137.

La Berge, Ann E. Fowler. *Mission and Method: The Early Nineteenth-Century French Public Health Movement.* Cambridge: Cambridge University Press, 1992.

Larson, Edward J. *Sex, Race, and Science: Eugenics in the Deep South.* Baltimore: Johns Hopkins University Press, 1996.

McKeown, Thomas, and C. R. Lowe. *An Introduction to Social Medicine.* Oxford: Blackwell Scientific, 1974.

Nathanson, Constance A. *Disease Prevention as Social Change The State, Society, and Public Health in the United States, France, Great Britain, and Canada*. New York: Russell Sage Foundation, 2007.

Nielsen, Waldemar A. *The Big Foundations*. New York: Columbia University Press, 1972.

Nowaczewska, Renata. *Dobroczynna Ameryka*. Warsaw: Warsaw University Press, 2009.

Pitt, Joseph. "Observations on the Country and Diseases near Roanoke River, in the State of North-Carolina." *New York Medical Repository* 5 (1808): 340-1.

Rockefeller Foundation, *The Annual Report of 1916*. New York, 1916.

—. *The Annual Report of 1917*. New York, 1917.

—. *The Annual Report of 1918*. New York, 1918.

—. *The Annual Report of 1920*. New York, 1920.

—. *The Annual Report of 1929*, New York, 1929.

—. International Health Board *Bibliography of Hookworm Disease*. Publ. No. 11, New York: IHB, 1922.

Rockefeller Archive Center, Sleepy Hollow, NY (RAC), Rockefeller Foundation, Excerpt from Trustees Bulletin, "Development of Rural Health Services," RG 3, Series 908, Box 14, File 149. December 1939. *100 Years: The Rockefeller Foundation*, accessed January 21, 2014, http://rockefeller100.org/items/show/2172.

RAC, Rockefeller Foundation, IHB/ Division records. "A Letter to John Ferrell" December 17, 1923, RG 5 Subseries 1.01: Correspondence, General 1910-1927, Box 69, Folder 971, The Rockefeller Archive Center, Sleepy Hollow, NY.

—. Rockefeller, John D., "Letter from John D. Rockefeller Sr. to Rockefeller Sanitary Commission board members, 1909 October 26," Office of the Messrs. Rockefeller Records, series O, Box 52, folder 544. *100 Years: The Rockefeller Foundation*, accessed January 22, 2014, http://rockefeller100.org/items/show/2162.

—. Rockefeller Foundation. "Preliminary Draft of Plan for Production of a Film on Hookworm Disease" Sept 12, 1917, RG 1.1, Series 100: International, 1913-1958, Box 5, Folder 42, *Films-Reports 1917-1927*.

—. Rockefeller Foundation, "Resolutions Establishing the International Health Commission," June 27, 1913. Administration, Program and Policy, RG 3.1, series 900, box 18, folder 129. *100 Years: The Rockefeller Foundation*, accessed January 22, 2014, http://rockefeller100.org/items/show/2159.

—. Rockefeller Foundation, IHB/ Division, "Tentative Scenario for Moving-Picture Film No. 2," RG 5, Series 1.2, Box 20, Folder 302, *938 – Films – General and Individual, 1914*.

—. Rockefeller Sanitary Commission for the Eradication of Hookworm Disease, "Letter from Rockefeller Sanitary Commission board members to John D. Rockefeller Sr., 1909 October 26," Office of the Messrs. Rockefeller records, series O, box 52, folder 544, *100 Years: The Rockefeller Foundation*, accessed January 25, 2014, http://rockefeller100.org/items/show/2162.

—. Rockefeller Sanitary Commission for the Eradication of Hookworm Disease records, Wickliffe Rose, "Work of the Rockefeller Sanitary Commission," August 13, 1914, series 1, box 2, folder 33, *100 Years: The Rockefeller Foundation*, accessed January 22, 2014, http://rockefeller100.org/items/show/1874.

—. "Unhooking the Hookworm." Accessed March 22, 2014. http://www.rockarch.org/feature/hookworm.php.

—. "Wickliffe Rose." Accessed March 22, 2014. http://rockefeller100.org/biography/show/wickliffe-rose

"Rockefeller Gift to Kill 'Hookworm': Million-Dollar Fund to Be Spent By a Commission." *New York Times* Oct 29, 1909, 1.

"The Rockefeller Report." *New York Times* (Nov 12, 1929): 29.

Savitt, Todd L. *Medicine and Slavery. The Diseases and Health Care of Blacks in Antebellum Virginia*. Urbana: University of Illinois Press, 1978.

Savitt, Todd L. and James H. Young. *Disease and Distinctiveness in the American South*. Knoxville: University of Tennessee Press, 1988.

Shaplen, Robert. *Toward the Well-Being of Mankind: Fifty Years of the Rockefeller Foundation*. Garden City, NY: Doubleday & Company, Inc., 1964.

Stiles, Ch. Wardell. *Report upon the Prevalence and Geographic Distribution of Hookworm Disease in the United States*. Washington: Government Printing Office, 1903.

—. "The Treatment of Hookworm Disease." *Public Health Reports* (1896-1970) 24, no. 34 (Aug. 20, 1909): 1191-1193.

Stiles, Ch. Wardell, and George F. Leonard. "Administration of Thymol in Hookworm Disease." *Public Health Reports* (1896-1970), 26(49), (Dec. 8, 1911): 1925.

The Tennessee Encyclopedia of History and Culture, "Wickliff Rose." Accessed March 22, 2014.
http://tennesseeencyclopedia.net/entry.php?rec=1150.

"To Study the Hookworm." *Chicago Daily* Tribune, October 30, 1909, 10.

Tullos, Allen. "The Germ of Laziness: Rockefeller Philanthropy and Public Health in the New South, by John Ettling, Harvard University Press, 1981. A Review." *The Journal of the Southern Regional Council* 4, no. 6 (1982): 15-17.

—. *Habits of Industry: White Culture and the Transformation of the Carolina Piedmont.* Chapel Hill: The University of North Carolina Press, 1989.

"Two Million Have Hookworm," *New York Times*, October 13, 1909.

Wray, Matt. *Not Quite White. White Trash and the Boundaries of Whiteness.* Durham and London: Duke University Press, 2006.

CHAPTER TWO

FLANNERY O'CONNOR'S "THE ENDURING CHILL" AS A MEDICAL TALE

MARCEL ARBEIT

Flannery O'Connor is one of the southern writers for whom health was not just a theme but a truly existentialist matter. Much has been written about her serious disease, lupus, that killed her father and, years later, her, but little attention has been paid to illnesses and diseases in her fiction. Her two stories, "A Stroke of Good Fortune" and "The Enduring Chill," in which the theme of health and illness is most prominent, have usually been interpreted as metaphorical tales in which diseases stand for a more general, social, moral or religious problem that should be fixed. However, another vital possibility opens when we read them as symbolic tales in which the transfer of meanings does not obscure the presence of real health problems: a disease can symbolize many things but still remains a disease to be cured.

"The Enduring Chill," from the collection *Everything That Rises Must Converge*, first published in *Harper's Bazaar* in July 1958, describes the health troubles of Asbury Fox, a would-be intellectual and writer who, after several bouts of a mysterious illness, returns from his exile in New York to die on his native farm, run by his overprotective mother. Instead, he receives a diagnosis which is serious but not terminal and, in addition to that, the Holy Ghost, or at least a vision of its descent, that he never cared for.

While mostly read as a theological story,[1] "The Enduring Chill" is primarily a story of physical and mental illness and the close connection

---

[1] Most interpretations of this story are theological and Ted Spivey even considers it as "probably the most theologically explicit of all of O'Connor's stories." See Spivey, *Flannery O'Connor: The Woman, the Thinker, the Visionary* (Macon, GA: Mercer University Press, 1995), 151.

between the two. The symptoms of both are meticulously depicted, their reasons are found and verified, and the therapy is suggested. Nevertheless, no healing process is shown and, under the circumstances, there is grave doubt as to whether the patient can be completely cured.

When Asbury arrived by train at Timberboro, where his mother was waiting to meet him, he realized "for the first time that he must look as ill as he was."[2] Seeing her ghastly look, he was "pleased that she should see death in his face at once."[3] Now, in his opinion, his mother would have to take him seriously at last and acknowledge him as an ill person; in the past he had been, for her, and even more for his sister, just a big lazy child pretending to be a writer but lacking talent.

According to his mother, the only illness Asbury had suffered from in the past was his artistic ambitions. Besides preventing him from seeing things straight and standing with his feet firmly on the ground, they gave him crazy ideas: for example, to study the habits and manners of two black farmhands, Randall and Morgan, for the play he intended to write. She considered the best cure for this condition a stay in the fresh air and manual work on the farm, for example in the dairy. From Asbury's point of view, the root of his present illness is not his imagination but the lack of it: the writer's block that he has never been able to overcome, and that has not allowed him to write anything except a long letter of complaint addressed to his mother which she is supposed to read only after his death. The writer's block, for which he blames his mother, prevents him from bringing to fruition any of his more public creative projects, starting with the play about blacks and another "half-dozen stationary plays" and ending with "his sketchy short stories."[4] Even his flight from the direct influence of his mother to the urban North did not help. Like at home, in New York his imagination is only "some bird" his mother "had domesticated, sitting huffy in its pen, refusing to come out!",[5] rather poultry than a bird of prey. Full of anxiety and despair, Asbury ends his letter with a twicc-underscored summary of his life: "I have no imagination. I have no talent. I can't create. I have nothing but the desire for these things. Why didn't you kill that too? Woman, why did you pinion me?"[6]

When Asbury was in New York, one of his friends took him to a lecture on Vedanta. Asbury found the lecture, filled also with Zen

---

[2] Flannery O'Connor, "The Enduring Chill," *The Complete Stories* (New York: Farrar, Straus and Giroux, 1971), 357.

[3] Ibid.

[4] Ibid., 365

[5] Ibid., 364.

[6] Ibid.

Buddhist truisms, extremely boring but noticed a Jesuit priest in black who shared his "taciturn superior expression."[7] The priest said that there was "a real probability of the New Man, assisted, of course, . . . by the Third Person of the Trinity,"[8] that is, the Holy Ghost. The name of the Jesuit is Ignatius Vogle and it is symptomatic that the stain on the ceiling that at the end of the story turns into the Holy Ghost has the shape of a bird ("der Vogel" in German).[9]

At that time, physical symptoms have already joined the mental ones: he was afflicted in his cold New York flat by "a chill one night, followed by a violent sweat that left the sheets soaking," preceded by "a gradual slackening of his energy and vague inconsistent aches and headaches."[10]

While his sister Mary George considers his illness psychosomatic, Asbury's nature immediately brings into his mind a terminal disease and, consequently, the approach of death. But instead of fear, he feels satisfaction: now he can punish his mother for her misunderstanding and seeming negligence of his problems, show her that her motherly care was destructive. The critics who approach the story from a religious point of view see Asbury in a similar way as his sister does: as a pretentious pseudo-intellectual who believes that "all he's going to be around here for the next fifty years is a decoration."[11] Even such a thoughtful scholar as Robert H. Brinkmeyer, Jr. reads the story as just another tale of an isolated artist who finally undergoes a spiritual transformation, and downplays the symptoms of his physical illness.[12]

Seen from the viewpoint of medical anthropology, there are several ways to look at symptoms such as Asbury's: Cecil G. Helman, the British author of *Culture, Health and Illness* (1984), distinguishes between the patient's perspective and the doctor's perspective. These perspectives can overlap when a patient is at the same time a doctor with a relevant specialization,[13] but Asbury is not a medical professional, and without his

---

[7] Ibid., 360.

[8] Ibid., 360.

[9] Numerous scholars have made a similar point: see, for example, Whitt, *Understanding Flannery O'Connor*, 133; Gentry, *Flannery O'Connor*, 51, and many others.

[10] Ibid., 358.

[11] Ibid., 373.

[12] See Robert H. Brinkmeyer, Jr., *The Art and Vision of Flannery O'Connor* (Baton Rouge: Louisiana University Press, 1989), 84.

[13] This frequently happens in the novels of another southern writer, Walker Percy. Doctors who are at the same time patients appear in *The Last Gentleman* (1966), *Love in the Ruins* (1971), and *The Thanatos Syndrome* (1991), as well as in Percy's unpublished early novel *The Gramercy Winner*.

having the proper knowledge to diagnose himself, his illness is primarily what he feels. Helman emphasizes that the "patient's perspective on ill health is usually part of a much wider conceptual model used to explain misfortune in general; within this model illness is only a specialized form of adversity"[14] and it is true in Asbury's case as well: Asbury believes that his illness is the consequence of the misfortune brought on him through his mother's constant interfering with his privacy.

Eric J. Cassell, who explored relationships between patients and doctors, explains that before people decide to see a doctor, they have a non-specified illness, while after a visit to a doctor's office, the illness becomes a disease: "Disease, then, is something an organ has; illness is something a man has."[15] But between the first symptoms and the consultation with a professional, there is a period when people talk about their health problems with their friends or members of their families and seek advice from them: Helman uses for this "lay, non-professional, non-specialist domain of society" the term "the popular sector."[16] The most important part of the popular sector is the family but, as Helman shows, its specific culture, which involves, among other things, behavioral codes, can be "either protective or pathogenic," depending on the context; in the latter case, we can speak about "culturogenic stress."[17] Helman also claims that in the family "the main providers of health care are women, usually mothers or grandmothers, who diagnose most common illnesses and treat them with the materials at hand."[18] Such domestic care might help to cure a common illness, usually clustered under the non-specific label of "a cold" or "a viral infection" but other times it can be counterproductive. For example, C. E. Elliott-Binns's field research showed that in spite of mothers' good intentions, of all lay advisors they gave the second worst

---

[14] Cecil G. Helman, *Culture, Health and Illness*, 5th edition (London: Hodder Arnold, 2007), 126.

[15] Eric J. Cassell, *The Healer's Art: A New Approach to the Doctor-Patient Relationship* (New York: Lippincott, 1976), 48.

[16] Helman, *Culture, Health and Illness*, 82.

[17] Ibid., 293.

[18] Ibid., 82. Helman wrongly attributes this observation to Noel J. Chrisman. Chrisman does write about the significant role of families as providers of lay medical advices but does not identify providers of domestic treatment. In opposition to what Helman claims, Chrisman found out that within their families ill people most often consulted their spouses. See "The Health Seeking Process: An Approach to the Natural History of Illness." *Culture, Medicine and Psychiatry* 1.4 (1977): 366.

medical advice, being less harmful in this point only than mothers-in-law.[19]

This is not the case of Asbury's mother, though. After Asbury's return Mrs. Fox notices at first the most overt and most general symptoms of her son's condition: even though he is only twenty-five, he seems to her "puffy and pale," "his left eye was bloodshot," and "his hair had receded tragically;"[20] even Asbury's older sister admits that "there *is* something the matter with him" and that he "looks a hundred years old,"[21] and later laconically states, "If I looked as bad as you do, . . . I'd go to the hospital."[22] Soon Mrs. Fox notices that Asbury becomes exhausted too easily and is hardly able to drag his two heavy suitcases first into the car and then to the family home. Instead of suggesting a domestic cure, she wisely advises a visit to Doctor Block, their family doctor. Asbury vehemently disdains this idea—"Don't you think if I'd wanted to go to a doctor I'd have gone up there where they have some good ones? Don't you know they have better doctors in New York?"[23]—but his mother does not give up and produces a trump: "He would take a personal interest in you . . . None of those doctors up there would take a personal interest in you."[24]

But Asbury does not want a doctor with a personal approach to him; in fact, he does not want any doctor. Like mothers over their sons, doctors have too much power over their patients: as Helman suggests, they "have the power to question or examine their patients, prescribe powerful and sometimes dangerous treatments or medication, and deprive certain people of their freedom and confine them to hospitals . . ."[25] It is also a matter of their discretion to "label their patients (sometimes permanently) as ill, incurable, malingering, hypochondriacal, or fully recovered."[26] It is impossible to ignore or fight the authority of both doctors and mothers but, while ill people can, at least in some cases, avoid doctors if they do not lose consciousness or are not diagnosed with a contagious disease that could be dangerous for their surroundings, those who live with their

---

[19] See C. P. Elliott-Binns, "An Analysis of Lay Medicine," *Journal of the Royal College of General Practitioners* 23 (1973): 257–58. According to his research, only the advice found in popular magazines is more harmful.
[20] O'Connor, "The Enduring Chill," 357.
[21] Ibid., 363, O'Connor's italics.
[22] Ibid., 365.
[23] Ibid., 359.
[24] Ibid., 359.
[25] Helman, *Culture, Health and Illness*, 94.
[26] Ibid., 95.

mother have absolutely no chance of escaping her influence. As Asbury admits, "It was not that she had ever forced her way on him. That had never been necessary. Her way had simply been the air he breathed and when at last he had found other air, he couldn't survive in it."[27]

As Helen S. Garson aptly notes, in O'Connor's stories "parents and children want and expect things of each other that can never be given."[28] This is also valid for the relationship between Asbury and his mother. Margaret Earley Whitt nicely characterizes Mrs. Fox as "the kind of character that lets her intellectual son have his say, but not necessarily his way."[29] O'Connor does not make it easy for the reader to decide whether Asbury's accusations against his mother are just poor excuses for his own incompetence, or have justifiable grounds. The third-person narrator she uses does not side with either the mother or the son, preferring to deal with them, as well as the less prominent characters in the story, from a comic distance. Still, for most of the story, Asbury is the focalizer through whom the events are seen; therefore readers get primarily his thoughts, while his mother's ruminations mostly concern Asbury's expected hostile reactions to every idea of hers.

There is no need to demonize Mrs. Fox, as Asbury does in his letter, but she can indeed be blamed for most of what her son is accusing her of. On the one hand, she paid for Asbury's college studies (this fact is downplayed in the story as the narrator never tells us what exactly he studied); on the other hand, she constantly treats him as a little boy who is not able to make his own decisions. Immediately after Asbury's arrival, Mrs. Fox advises him to take off his coat and Asbury responds with an angry "I'm old enough to know when I want to take my coat off!"[30] She did not manage to prevent Asbury from leaving home for New York, but at least she travels to check on him there and tries her best to make him loathe his new whereabouts and awaken his desire for home: "You wouldn't live like this at home."[31] Although Mrs. Fox tolerates Asbury's interest in writing and even defends him from his sister, suggesting that he has not published anything because "he might be writing a very *long*

---

[27] O'Connor, "The Enduring Chill," 364–65.
[28] Helen S. Garson, "Cold Comfort: Parents and Children in the Work of Flannery O'Connor," *Realist of Distances: Flannery O'Connor Revisited*, eds. Karl-Heinz Westarp and Jan Nordby Gretlund (Aarhus: Aarhus University Press, 1987), 113.
[29] Margaret Earley Whitt, *Understanding Flannery O'Connor* (Columbia: University of South Carolina Press, 1995), 132.
[30] O'Connor, "The Enduring Chill," 358.
[31] Ibid., 362.

book,"[32] she never forgets to stress that, unlike manual labor on the farm such as working in the dairy or fixing fences, writing is not "real work."[33] Even these who give Mrs. Fox her due as a caring and conscientious woman, who, as a widow, combines the comforting role of a mother with the protective role of a father, must admit, as Richard Giannone does, that she did "an inadequate job of preparing Asbury for life," which includes "her not teaching her child his daily prayers,"[34] as Father Finn, the Jesuit whom Asbury makes his mother invite for a conversation, immediately recognizes. One of the black farmhands, Randall, is even more radical in this matter: "She ain't whup him enough when he was little."[35]

Even though it is always tricky to read a story through its author's life, it is obvious that the character of Mrs. Fox is modeled after O'Connor's mother Regina, whom O'Connor described to her friend Maryat Lee as "mayor, sheriff, judge, treasurer and boss of this little state—a feudal state where she was feudal queen."[36] The same can be said about mothers in her other stories, but in this case some plot elements copy real life.[37] Not only did O'Connor return home from the North because of her disease and, as in Asbury's case, her stay on the family farm became permanent, but even Regina's comments on her writing resemble those of Mrs. Fox. While Mrs. Fox advises Asbury to write "a book about down here . . . another good book like *Gone With the Wind*,"[38] in one of her letters to Cecil Dawkins, a teacher and writer from Alabama, O'Connor describes a similar piece of advice from Regina: "Do you think, she said, that you are really using the talent God gave you when you don't write something that a lot, a LOT, of people like?"[39] Such well-meant advice from a loving parent can cause a major mental problem, accompanied by a physical response of the body, which O'Connor aptly illustrates in the same letter:

---

[32] Ibid., 363, O'Connor's italics.
[33] Ibid., 361.
[34] Richard Giannone, *Flannery O'Connor and the Mystery of Life* (New York: Fordham University Press, 1999), 188.
[35] O'Connor, "The Enduring Chill," 370.
[36] Jean W. Cash, *Flannery O'Connor: A Life* (Knoxville: University of Tennessee Press, 2002), 237. Maryat Lee cites it in her journal entry written after O'Connor's death, in early 1965.
[37] Multiple pieces of evidence are given in the chapter "Regina and Flannery" in Cash, 145–73. Compare especially the arguments on page 171.
[38] O'Connor, "The Enduring Chill," 370.
[39] Flannery O'Connor, *The Habit of Being*, ed. Sally Fitzgerald (New York: Farrar, Straus and Giroux, 1979), 326.

"This always leaves me shaking and speechless, raises my blood pressure 140 degrees, etc."[40]

Asbury does not seek a diagnosis or a cure. His desire is to overpower his mother; her helplessness in the face of his grave condition would be the most efficient blow he could deal her. Asbury's twice-repeated statement "What's wrong with me is way beyond Block"[41] nevertheless shows how unintentionally close his idea that the illness of his body, even though physical, resulted from the troubles of his mind, is to his mother's opinion that his condition is an incipient "nervous breakdown."[42] Mrs. Fox's idea follows the commonsense logic that finds support in numerous medical research studies: there is evidence that, as Helman shows, "individuals with psychiatric disorders" have "a significantly higher rate of organic illness," and among the most powerful stressors are "a feeling of psychological impotence or helplessness" and "a lowered self-image as one who is no longer competent, in control or functioning in the usual manner."[43] Asbury's symptoms, especially the regularly alternating fever and chills, could be signals of stress which triggers a somatic response.

When in the afternoon Asbury finds out that his mother has responded to his unwillingness to visit Dr. Block by inviting the doctor to their house, he becomes furious, as he finds himself squeezed by their double power. Mrs. Fox tries to organize Asbury's day and decides when he is supposed to sit on the porch and enjoy the sunshine and when he should sleep. According to Helman, illness "creates a temporary caring community around the victim, and old antagonisms are forgotten, at least for the moment,"[44] but in this case only the first part of this statement applies, as not only are the grudges between mother and son still alive but they even escalate.

Dr. Block, who is a general practitioner for most, if not all, of the families in the local community, is well aware of the interconnection of the popular sector with the professional one in the healing process. He also keeps in mind the southern tradition of the intermediary "folk sector" of healers, herbalists and shamans, both sacred and secular, who, lacking formal medical education but possessing great psychological skills, helped their patients substantially, using an approach that modern medical anthropology calls holistic, "dealing with *all* aspects of the patient's

---

[40] Ibid., 326.
[41] O'Connor, "The Enduring Chill," 359, 360.
[42] Ibid., 360.
[43] Helman, *Culture, Health and Illness*, 291–92.
[44] Ibid., 240.

life."[45] As Helman points out, for the healers in the folk sector health "is seen as a *balance* between people and their social, natural and supernatural environments," and that is why their methods include the close examination of "the patient's behavior before the illness"[46] and the "involvement of the family in diagnosis and treatment."[47]

On the one hand, Dr. Block is a clown-like figure who makes "a face like a Chinaman," rolling his eyes "almost out of his head" and even "wiggling his ears;"[48] on the other hand, he has "two cold clinical nickel-colored eyes that hung with a motionless curiosity over whatever he looked at."[49] It corresponds to his double identity as a folk healer and a scientist. His funny faces are the lure for his child patients, who might be scared by a strict and serious doctor in a white coat but will obey a friendly elderly man with a pink face and large ears. Local children sometimes even "vomited and went into fevers to have a visit from him"[50] but the twenty-five-year-old Asbury welcomes the doctor with open hostility. Asbury rejects Dr. Block's folk healer identity, as it makes him an ally of his mother, who behaves "as if she had captured this angel on the rooftop and brought him in for her little boy,"[51] as well as his identity as a professional, as it could invalidate Asbury's lay prognosis of early death.

The first observation of Dr. Block fully corresponds with Asbury's perception of himself and his condition. When Asbury entered the house, he paused in the hall to see "his pale broken face glare at him" in a pier mirror;[52] now Dr. Block confirms what the mirror showed with his inexorable "I don't know when I've seen anybody your age look as sorry as you do."[53] Trying to delay the moment when his unspecified illness becomes a disease, he snaps shut his mouth, which he automatically opens when Dr. Block orders him to "Say AHHHH!",[54] but then the doctor takes his blood and a decisive step toward a proper diagnosis is made because, in Dr. Block's words, "Blood don't lie."[55]

---

[45] Ibid., 85, Helman's italics.
[46] Ibid., 85, Helman's italics.
[47] Ibid., 87. Among those, who rely exclusively on the folk sector for a cure, are the two black farmhands, Randall and Morgan; when Morgan has a cold, he takes "a little turpentine and sugar" (O'Connor, "The Enduring Chill," 380).
[48] O'Connor, "The Enduring Chill," 366.
[49] Ibid.
[50] Ibid.
[51] Ibid.
[52] Ibid., 363.
[53] Ibid., 366.
[54] Ibid.
[55] Ibid., 367.

Dr. Block and Mrs. Fox, who does not speak about a nervous breakdown any more, side with each other in their effort to cure Asbury's physical illness, at the same time ignoring the illness of his mind triggered by his mother's inability to see his desire to be an artist as little more than a foolish whim. Mrs. Fox does not believe in the power of Art, but she trusts the current progress of medical science and the people who represent it: "Nowadays doctors don't *let* young people die. They give them some of these new medicines. . . . People just don't die like they used to."[56] She thinks that Asbury's ugly behavior towards Dr. Block proves that he is "really sick,"[57] but the final evidence that the illness is "a real disease" is in the fact that the "doctor says so."[58]

As stated earlier, Asbury, who realized that he had no talent or future, does not crave recovery but a chance to hurt his mother. He takes his seemingly approaching death as his "greatest triumph" that will launch his mother's "private revelation," even though he prefers death "coming to him legitimately" to its most spectacular form, suicide. His suicide "would indicate a mother who had been a failure," which is exactly what he thinks, but at the same time expose her to "a public embarrassment,"[59] which, in his opinion, would be too harsh a punishment for her. Although Asbury constantly snaps at his mother, he cannot ignore her newly-born interest in his creative activities, even though it is naïve, clumsy and long overdue: she offers him the chance "to have a little studio" in his room[60] and encourages him to write a long novel with the Civil War in it. In the light of her previous stance toward his artistic inclinations, Asbury interprets her changed approach as true evidence of his serious condition. The behavior of Dr. Block, who "looked now as if he knew he was battling the real thing," together with the "first distinct stroke of doubt" in his mother's eyes, supports the explanation that Mrs. Fox simply wanted to please her dying son: "He looked like one of those dying children who must have Christmas early."[61]

Subjectively, Asbury's condition really got worse and new symptoms—increased debilitation and a want of appetite—joined the old ones: "his fever had increased, interspersed by chills; he barely had the energy to drag himself out on the porch; food was abhorrent to him. . . . Even as he sat there, he felt the beginning of a new chill, as if death were already

[56] Ibid., 372, O'Connor's italics.
[57] Ibid., 367.
[58] Ibid., 373.
[59] Ibid., 370.
[60] Ibid., 365.
[61] Ibid., 372, 374.

playfully rattling his bones."[62] Feeding the image of himself as a dying man whose future is "the peaceful spot in the family burying ground," he dreams about his body being carried toward the graveyard, while "his mother and Mary George watched without interest from their chairs on the porch."[63] This picturesque image, complete with the dark figure of a Jesuit priest following the procession and "a shallow grave on the hillside and the indistinct mourners," ends with a "violently spotted" cow that is "softly licking his head as if it were a block of salt."[64] The pastoral idyll at the end of his dream is in sharp contrast with the gloominess of his daily ruminations; his suppressed creativity shows only when he sleeps, while during his waking hours, Art with a capital "A" is only "sending him Death."[65]

Storytellers, and not only southern ones, usually outlive their biological death through their stories; their social death comes only when the stories are forgotten. To postpone their social death, people do not even have to be the narrators of the tales; it is enough to be their subjects. Asbury considers himself to be socially dead but there are some stories with him as a protagonist that rest in his mother's memory, for example the story about his work in the dairy that ended when a cow kicked him. Even such stories of failure form Asbury's personal identity and may prolong his existence after his body dies.[66]

After the visit of Father Finn, Asbury looks so "pale and drawn and ravaged"[67] that his mother considers taking him to a hospital. As a southerner who grew up on his mother's farm, Asbury is understandably scared to lose even the most basic identity he has, the one consisting of his name and family, as well as his community roots. Even though he despises

---

[62] Ibid., 372.
[63] Ibid., 373–74.
[64] Ibid., 374.
[65] Ibid., 373.
[66] Influenced by Robert Hertz, the French philosopher and sociologist, Helman distinguishes between two types of death: one is biological and "is the end of the human organism" and the other is social and "is the end of the person's social identity" (Helman, 231). In his essay "Contribution à une étude sur représentation collective de la mort" ("A Contribution to the Study of the Collective Representation of Death," 1904, published in 1907), Hertz takes death as "a temporary exclusion of the individual from human society" that "effects his passage from the visible society of the living into the invisible society of the dead." See Hertz, *Death & the Right Hand*, trans. Rodney Needham and Claudia Needham (Glencoe, IL: Free Press, 1960), 86. On the other hand, Asbury believes that his social death has preceded his biological one, which increases his anxiety.
[67] O'Connor, "The Enduring Chill," 377.

his late father and blames his mother for his failures, he does not want to be completely depersonalized, "converted into a numbered 'case' in a ward full of strangers," as Helman describes the transition from everyday life to the life in what he calls, inspired by the sociologist Victor Turner, "a community of suffering."[68] According to Helman, hospital patients lose "control over one's body, and over personal space, privacy, behavior, diet and use of time," being "stripped of many of the props of social identity and individuality, and clothed in a uniform of pyjamas, nightdress or bathrobe."[69] Paradoxically, Asbury would never allow himself to be taken to a hospital while conscious because of the fear that they might cure him there, "fill him full of blood and prolong his misery for days."[70]

A transfusion would be the worst threat to Asbury's identity: then his blood would not be really his. Even Dr. Block's series of diagnostic blood tests is an invasion into "the privacy of his blood"[71]—both metaphorically, as visible blood traditionally means transition, for example from life to death in the case of a mortal wound, and literally, as the blood finally does tell the truth and identifies the real nature of Asbury's mysterious illness, which now acquires the contours of a specific disease, undulating fever, similar to Bang's (or Bang) disease in cows. Caused by "the bacteria of the genus Brucella," it is spread in humans through contact with contaminated animals or animal products; its symptoms "are similar to the flu and may include fever, sweats, headaches, back pains, and physical weakness."[72] If not treated, which was the case of Asbury, who was diagnosed with brucellosis approximately one year after he was infected,[73] the symptoms become chronic and include "recurrent fevers, joint pain, and fatigue," and, which is especially relevant for the analysis of this story, "depressive episodes."[74]

Asbury contracted the disease through drinking unpasteurized milk a year earlier. His reason for this irresponsible deed was to show his

---

[68] Helman, *Culture, Health and Illness*, 99, 84.
[69] Ibid., 99.
[70] O'Connor, "The Enduring Chill," 377.
[71] Ibid., 367.
[72] James N. Parker and Philip M. Parker, eds., *The Official Patient's Sourcebook on Brucellosis* (San Diego: ICON Group International, 2002), 10–11. According to this source, the acute form comes less than eight weeks after the contamination, followed by the undulant form, and developing after one year into the chronic form, which can include arthritis and, in less than 5% of patients, acute neurological symptoms.
[73] Giannone and others give the duration of Asbury's illness as only four months, forgetting the much earlier unspecific symptoms. See, for example, Giannone, 185.
[74] Parker and Parker, eds., *The Official Patient's Sourcebook on Brucellosis*, 14.

disobedience to his mother in the presence of her two black farmhands. Unlike his earlier protest against his mother's authority, when he had persuaded the two blacks to smoke in the dairy, this time the farmhands refused to join him in drinking the milk even though Asbury tried to make out that this transgression of the rules was a bonding ritual: the blacks only repeated "She don't 'low it,"[75] knowing that Mrs. Fox's ban must have had good reasons.[76]

The fact that Asbury suffered from a cattle disease has not escaped the attention of O'Connor scholars. For several of them, it was a punishment for his negligent approach to cows, the cattle that his mother was breeding. Whitt, alluding to the lecture on Vedanta Asbury attended in New York, takes as an irony that it is "the cow, the sacred animal to the Hindu" that "is later determined to be the source of Asbury's undulant fever."[77] Jill Peláez Baumgaertner, referring to another scene with cows, the one in which Asbury gets angry when his mother stops her car to examine a sick cow and, in the next moment, he must face a steady look from "a small, walleyed Guernsey,"[78] was even blunter in connecting Asbury's illness with these even-toed undulates. Having exclaimed "Good God!"[79] Asbury took "God's name in vain" and, as God is in cows (Baumgaertner does not claim they are sacred), "it is through this infection from cow's milk that God will finally be able to reach Asbury."[80] Considering, moreover,

---

[75] O'Connor, "The Enduring Chill," 370.

[76] Ralph C. Wood even thought that the blacks had known about the dangers of drinking unpasteurized milk and had not warned Asbury on purpose. See Wood, *Flannery O'Connor and the Christ-Haunted South* (Grand Rapids, MI: William B. Eerdmans, 2004), 115. On the other hand, Helen S. Garson believes that Mrs. Fox had no idea about the possibility of contracting a disease this way, "not knowing the scientific reasons," which, in my opinion, is very difficult to believe as she was a lifelong farmer and the narrator of the story does not make sure that she knew about this particular breach of the rules by Asbury. See Helen S. Garson, "Cold Comfort," 120.

[77] Whitt, *Understanding Flannery O'Connor*, 133. In this context, she also noticed that the name of Goetz, Asbury's friend who had invited him to the lecture, was derived from a German diminutive for God.

[78] O'Connor, "The Enduring Chill," 362.

[79] Ibid., 362.

[80] Jill Peláez Baumgaertner, *Flannery O'Connor: A Proper Scaring*, rev. ed. (Chicago: Cornerstone Press, 1999), 107. The quotation from O'Connor is, of course, ambiguous: the cow can bring Asbury to a belief in God, or, through its milk, it can make his punishment easier for God, or the milk can even kill Asbury and thus hasten his meeting with his Maker. Baumgaertner considers the first two

Asbury's dream about the cow licking his head, it would also be possible to blame cows for his writer's block, even though Asbury suffered from it before he drank a single drop of the harmful liquid.[81]

Those who consider cows, rather than unpasteurized milk, the source of Asbury's illness, see the disease as primarily social, which is typical of the folk sector, as Helman writes. Even if we rule out the theory of a revenge of sacred cows, according to folk tradition, animals, like human sorcerers or witches, can lay a curse on people; then, from such a point of view, the gazing little Guernsey could have given Asbury the evil eye.[82] From the medical perspective, Asbury's brucellosis is a curse only metaphorically, yet the disease was not an easy-to-cure one in 1957, nor even now. First, Brucella "can affect a number of different tissues," even though it is "most typically associated with the lympho-histiocytic disease," a disease caused by over-production of white blood cells, which "if left untreated invades other tissues and can kill the host," and, second, even after a successful treatment "relapse is not uncommon."[83] Mrs. Fox speaks about "some of these new medicines,"[84] that is, antibiotics, but at the time when the story was written their use was limited.[85]

---

options, finally giving preference to the first one, because of the emergence of yet another block on Asbury's path, Dr. Block.

[81] Marshall Bruce Gentry offers the opposite interpretation of Asbury's dream about the cow that licked him; in his opinion, it proves an unconscious desire for "some connection to the physical life of the farm community." Gentry, claiming that Asbury subconsciously never wanted to leave home, can nevertheless hardly find any proof for his interpretation in O'Connor's text. See Gentry, *Flannery O'Connor's Religion of the Grotesque* (Jackson: University Press of Mississippi, 1986), 51. See also Giannone, 190–93.

[82] For more about such beliefs and healers responding to them see Helman, 85.

[83] James N. Parker, and Philip M. Parker, eds., *Brucellosis: A Medical Dictionary, Bibliography, and Annotated Research Guide to Internet References* (San Diego: ICON Group International, 2004), 8. In the plan of the research project "Improved Brucella Vaccine Strains," performed at Texas A & M University in the years 2001–04, the team points out the difficulties with the development of a safe and reliable vaccine and, with a growing antibiotic resistance to Brucella, the treatment becomes even more complicated. For basically identical information, see also James N. Parker and Philip M. Parker, eds., *The Official Patient's Sourcebook on Brucellosis*, 37–38.

[84] O'Connor, "The Enduring Chill," 372.

[85] Of the three antibiotics that are most commonly used for the treatment of brucellosis, only streptomycin was available at the time when the story was written, and the combined six-week use of rifampin and doxycycline, which is usually prescribed these days, could not be used, as rifampin (also known as rifampicin) was produced for the first time in 1959 and doxycycline was developed

There is a significant irony in the fact that Asbury's physical symptoms prove to have nothing to do with his mental problems: the opinion of Asbury's sister that "Asbury can't write so he gets sick"[86] and that several shock treatments would cure him turns out to be wrong. On the other hand, the lay belief which is typical of the modern Western world, i.e., that "the *responsibility* for illness falls mainly. . . on the patients themselves,"[87] comes true in Asbury's case.

That is why the cures for his body and soul must come from different directions. During his illness Asbury feels "as if he were a shell that had to be filled with something but he did not know what,"[88] even though on the previous day Father Finn, the old Jesuit priest, blind in one eye and deaf in one ear, showed him a way: in his opinion, Asbury should ask God to send the Holy Ghost, as "God does not send the Holy Ghost to those who don't ask for Him."[89] To Asbury's angry reaction that the Holy Ghost "is the last thing" he is looking for, Father Finn calmly replies: "And He may be the last thing you get."[90] Before his exit, the priest further adds, "The Holy Ghost will not come until you see yourself as you are—a lazy ignorant conceited youth!"[91] The old priest does plant a seed into Asbury's mind, as the following morning Asbury finds himself "thinking of his useless life."[92]

The climax and at the same time the dénouement of the story, that is, the descent of the Holy Ghost into Asbury, can be read in several ways. Symbolically, the Holy Ghost, having assumed the image of a water stain on the ceiling, shaped like "a fierce bird with spread wings" with "an icicle crosswise in its beak" and "smaller icicles depending from its wings and tail,"[93] has been waiting since Asbury's childhood to be invited, but the sight of him has so far made Asbury irritated or frightened. The disease makes Asbury weak and unable to fight any more: when he feels that the stain has finally moved, only a "feeble cry, a last impossible protest

---

in the early 1960s and approved in the U.S. as late as 1967. See Parker, and Parker, *Brucellosis*, 13. The source attributes less than 2% mortality to the disease, but only when it is treated properly.

86 O'Connor, "The Enduring Chill," 373.

87 Helman, *Culture, Health and Illness*, 104, Helman's italics.

88 O'Connor, "The Enduring Chill," 377–78.

89 Ibid., 376.

90 Ibid.

91 Ibid., 377.

92 Ibid.

93 Ibid., 365.

escaped him,"[94] which is of no avail, as the image, the Holy Ghost, is getting nearer and nearer. The descent of the Holy Ghost is not a prayer of Asbury's that has been answered or the fulfillment of his secret wish. In agreement with the medical context of the story, it is a scene in which a virus penetrates a weakened body, or, contrary to that, a scene in which a medicine is administered to a patient against his will.

However, most interpreters of the story missed the irony of the conclusion and consider Asbury just another O'Connor character receiving grace. What I take as a loss of Asbury's defenses as a result of his disease, others see as a logical ending of the subconscious quest for God that Asbury embarked on when, as a child, he noticed the stain for the first time. Frederick Asals, for example, takes Asbury's willpower as the main obstacle to his artistic imagination, and in the loss of his free will, which, in the past, led him to futile challenges of "a reality greater than itself" he sees "the release of Asbury's stifled imagination."[95] Nevertheless, the question still lingers as to whether Asbury's ability to recognize the descending Holy Ghost in a bird-shaped water stain is evidence of his finally having acquired an artistic vision, or just another symptom of his disease.

But even if we accept the theological interpretation, the ending of the story remains ambiguous. In the New Testament, Jesus, while staying with the Apostles, told them not to leave Jerusalem and wait for baptism "with the Holy Spirit not many days from now."[96] On the day of Pentecost,

> suddenly from heaven there came a sound like the rush of a violent wind, and it filled the entire house where they were sitting. Divided tongues, as of fire, appeared among them, and a tongue rested on each of them. All of them were filled with the Holy Spirit and began to speak in other languages, as the Spirit gave them ability.[97]

It is doubtful whether Asbury would profit from the ability to speak in other languages, as in all these languages Lord's sons and daughters should prophesy "the coming of the Lord's great and glorious day,"[98] while Asbury does not know his catechism, his mother "doesn't have time

---

[94] Ibid., 382.
[95] Frederick Asals, *Flannery O'Connor: The Imagination of Extremity* (1982; Athens: University of Georgia Press, 2007), 125, 224.
[96] Acts 1:5.
[97] Acts 2:2–4.
[98] Acts 2:20.

to pray" and his sister is an atheist.[99] According to the Scriptures, "young men shall see visions,"[100] but Asbury's vision is not the Biblical one of the sun "turned to darkness and the moon to blood;"[101] for him it is even more awful, a contrary vision of a "blinding red-gold sun" moving "serenely from under a purple cloud."[102] Asbury is helplessly awaiting the coming of a new life: "He saw that for the rest of his days, frail, racked, but enduring, he would live in the face of a purifying terror."[103] Brinkmeyer considers this an epiphany, as well as a result of several of Asbury's failures in communication: Asbury is not able to have a proper conversation either with the black farmhands or with Father Finn, and he "fails even in his plans for death." Dr. Block's diagnosis that sentences him to life (the ambiguity of the phrase is fitting) shocks him, in Brinkmeyer's opinion, "into seeing himself as he truly is— vain and pretentious, with no one to blame for his errors except himself."[104] But the ending of the story does not suggest in the least that Asbury takes all the blame on himself. Even though "the last film of illusion" is really "torn as if by a whirlwind from his eyes,"[105] this descend into a vortex only makes him, instead of a creator of art, its humiliated object.[106] The purifying terror the narrator refers to is the existential *angst* of a man who faces not only a life without a creative talent—this he found out long ago—but also a life with a disease about which he is not told anything but that he "ain't going to die," even though it will "keep coming back."[107]

Asbury nevertheless realizes that one authority that made him a slave, his mother, was joined by another one, infinitely more powerful and, hopefully, less malign. It can hardly be guessed whether Asbury would

---

[99] O'Connor, "The Enduring Chill," 376.
[100] Acts 2:17.
[101] Acts 2:20.
[102] O'Connor, "The Enduring Chill," 382.
[103] Ibid.
[104] Brinkmeyer, Jr., *The Art and Vision of Flannery O'Connor*, 87.
[105] O'Connor, "The Enduring Chill," 382.
[106] On the one hand, O'Connor alludes here to Ezra Pound's vorticism, the poetic style admired by her "erstwhile boy friends" who "visit Pound . . . and think he is made and finished—he calls them all funny names and they think its (*sic*) wonderful, touched by the holy hand, etc" (O'Connor, *The Habit of Being*, 132). On the other hand, Asbury becomes an armchair version of the brave but irresponsible fisherman from Edgar Allan Poe's "A Descent Into the Maelström," who after his encounter with "gigantic and innumerable vortices" looks like "a traveller from the spirit-land." See Poe, "A Descent Into the Maelström," *Poetry and Tales* (New York: Library of America, 1984), 434, 448.
[107] Ibid., 381.

become a real artist without the stifling influence of his mother, but it is sure that Mrs. Fox can be rightfully blamed for his brucellosis, as she never told him why he should not drink fresh milk in the dairy; like the two blacks who work for her and whom she treats as inferior, he is supposed to simply obey her orders and not to ask questions. There is an irony again: Asbury wants to leave his mother with "an enduring chill"[108] through his accusatory letter; instead, she gives him the chill by not providing him with a proper warning. In other words, as George A. Kilcourse, Jr. sums it up, the "effect he intends the letter to have on his mother backfires."[109] Contracting a cattle disease, for his mother Asbury becomes one of the ill cows of her herd, like the one "with a bad quarter"[110] that she spotted when she was driving Asbury home from the railway station.

Mrs. Fox behaves like a minor god, the one whom "he didn't know" in the very first paragraph of the story and whose temple the small decayed town of Timberboro became in his short vision of a forthcoming "majestic transformation."[111] The transformation really happened, but the one who was transformed was not the town but he himself. The agents of his transformation were his mother, his disease, and the God of all Christians. Mrs. Fox, who possesses a savior complex, asks Asbury, who, with malicious joy, is preparing her for his death: "Do you think for one minute . . . that I intend to sit here and let you die?"[112] Like God, Mr. Fox does not offer explanations, or give reasons for her acts, but when it comes to deeds, she becomes helpless in comparison with the Almighty.[113]

Asbury is equally helpless when he faces the Holy Ghost at the end of the story, a man not at the threshold of death as he thought to be, but on the verge of losing his free will. The ending is a spiritual awakening upside down: instead of darkness there is a blazing light, instead of rejoicing, terror, and, instead of warmth, a chill. The Holy Ghost, "emblazoned in ice instead of fire,"[114] which came from a stain on the

[108] Ibid., 365.
[109] George A. Kilcourse, Jr., *Flannery O'Connor's Religious Imagination: A World with Everything Off Balance* (New York; Mahwah, NJ: Paulist Press, 2001), 260.
[110] O'Connor, "The Enduring Chill," 362.
[111] Ibid., 357.
[112] Ibid., 372.
[113] Brinkmeyer writes about "a severe commitment to an all-demanding God," (88) but for him the commitment is not that of Asbury but that of O'Connor, whom he joins with the narrator of the story. Considering the role of the author in the narrative, Asbury does not seem to be just a target of irony and criticism.
[114] O'Connor, "The Enduring Chill," 382.

ceiling, might save Asbury's soul but whether He can cure his mental problems is doubtful: do people living in "a purifying terror" get rid of all their anxieties? Even if the Holy Ghost is the last thing Asbury might get, as Father Finn ominously told him, it is impossible to guess how long "the rest of his days" will be. Both a virus and a remedy, the Holy Ghost from Asbury's vision brings him to an acknowledgment of God and His power, if not, for the time being, a belief in Him, and at the same time dilutes Asbury's damaging dependence on his mother: from now he will have a new master whom he will use against the old one. His mother was irritated by Asbury's wish to talk to a Jesuit priest, objecting that he is "not a member of that church"[115] and Asbury can expect that even a possibility of his true belief in God would upset her even more. In addition to that, the faith would alleviate the psychological pressure on him, as religious people are more immune to mental diseases; they can reduce anxiety and stress by adopting the view "of misfortune as being an expression of divine will or fate,"[116] while Asbury's earlier stance—the laying of the blame for his creative incompetence on his mother's shoulders—was closer to a pagan approach according to which people could be hexed by a person, not excluding family members.

In a letter to "A." [Betty Hester] from 28 December 1957, O'Connor wrote on Asbury: "So I have let it be known that he undeniably realizes that he's going to live with the new knowledge that he knows nothing. That really is what he is frozen in—humility. Faith can come later."[117] That is also why she planned to return to the characters of this story and invent a broader narrative context for them.[118] The question of whether the recognized presence of the Holy Ghost also means faith for Asbury is not sufficiently answered in the story but it does not make it any worse; on the contrary, its comic ambiguities add much value to the narrative, even though O'Connor herself voiced a different opinion.

Too much stress on health and illness might have been the reason why O'Connor continued to be haunted by the characters in it and considered a rewriting of the story to the last days of her life.[119] Criticized by Allen Tate

---

[115] Ibid., 371.
[116] Helman, *Culture, Health and Illness*, 293.
[117] O'Connor, *The Habit of Being*, 261.
[118] Ibid., 546. O'Connor suggests it, for example, in a letter to Cecil Dawkins, who was writing a full-length play based on her short stories and wanted to use the characters of Asbury and Father Finn in his work. In the letter, dated 5 November 1963, O'Connor did not want Dawkins to use these characters.
[119] Even as late as 28 June 1964 she wrote to Robert Giroux, the publisher of her second collection of stories, that she plans "considerable rewriting" of the story

and Caroline Gordon for introducing the Holy Ghost too late,[120] she adopted this criticism as her own and in an August 1958 letter to her friend Maryat Lee she wrote: "The problem was to have the Holy Ghost descend by degrees throughout the story but unrecognized, but at the end recognized, coming down, implacable, with ice instead of fire."[121] Her *ex post* plans at making the story even more theological than medical—fortunately, never realized—became even more obvious after she met a reader who thought that Asbury had died in the end: "Because the bird began to move down, the person seemed to think Asbury started to move up."[122] From a medical perspective, such a reading of the story is not so preposterous: the descent of the Holy Ghost could be interpreted as a delusion of the dying Asbury, whose mind materialized Father Finn's prophecy about the Holy Ghost being the last thing he gets.

Asbury's peculiar conversion, even if not a product of his delusional mind, cannot cure his body, as his brucellosis, discovered too late not to turn into its second, undulant, or even third, chronic phase, is cyclical and Asbury will suffer from it until he dies. Asbury's confinement on his mother's farm in the company of his bitter and cynical sister makes this comic story one of the saddest and at the same time most chilling in O'Connor's literary canon. When read as a theological story, "The Enduring Chill" may have some flaws, but as a medical story it is an exemplary and merciless examination, by a skillful practitioner, of the condition and health not only of its main protagonist, but also of family relationships and, last but not least, human faith.

(O'Connor, *The Habit of Being*, 589), but finally she decided against it: in *The Collected Stories* it was published exactly as it appeared in *Harper's Bazaar*. As she admits in a letter to Catharine Carver dated 15 July 1964, she was afraid that she might "make it worse than it is" (O'Connor, *The Habit of Being*, 593).

[120] See O'Connor, *The Habit of Being*, 261.

[121] Ibid., 293. Edward Kessler, using basically the same facts, comes to the conclusion that O'Connor "strained to will it [the story] into a theological concept" and "deserted the ambiguity central to metaphor for the certainties of direct statement." See Kessler, *Flannery O'Connor and the Language of Apocalypse* (Princeton, NJ: Princeton University Press, 1986), 128. Unlike Kessler, I read the ending as ambiguous, the source of the ambiguity being the tension between the theological and medical interpretation of the story.

[122] O'Connor, *The Habit of Being*, 372.

Works Cited

Asals, Frederick. *Flannery O'Connor: The Imagination of Extremity.* 1982. Athens: University of Georgia Press, 2007.

Baumgaertner, Jill Peláez. *Flannery O'Connor: A Proper Scaring.* Revised edition. Chicago: Cornerstone Press, 1999.

Brinkmeyer, Robert H., Jr. *The Art & Vision of Flannery O'Connor.* Baton Rouge: Louisiana State University Press, 1989.

Cash, Jean W. *Flannery O'Connor: A Life.* Knoxville: University of Tennessee Press, 2002.

Chrisman, Noel J. "The Health Seeking Process: An Approach to the Natural History of Illness." *Culture, Medicine and Psychiatry* 1.4 (1977): 351–77.

Elliott-Binns, C. P. "An Analysis of Lay Medicine." *Journal of the Royal College of General Practitioners* 23 (1973): 255–64.

Garson, Helen S. "Cold Comfort: Parents and Children in the Work of Flannery O'Connor." In *Realist of Distances: Flannery O'Connor Revisited,* edited by Karl-Heinz Westarp and Jan Nordby Gretlund. Aarhus: Aarhus University Press, 1987. 113–22.

Gentry, Marshall Bruce. *Flannery O'Connor's Religion of the Grotesque.* Jackson: University Press of Mississippi, 1986.

Giannone, Richard. *Flannery O'Connor and the Mystery of Life.* New York: Fordham University Press, 1999.

Helman, Cecil G. *Culture, Health and Illness.* 5th edition. London: Hodder Arnold, 2007.

Hertz, Robert. *Death & the Right Hand,* translated by Rodney Needham and Claudia Needham. Glencoe, IL: Free Press, 1960.

Kessler, Edward. *Flannery O'Connor and the Language of Apocalypse.* Princeton, NJ: Princeton University Press, 1986.

Kilcourse, George A., Jr. *Flannery O'Connor's Religious Imagination: A World with Everything Off Balance.* New York; Mahwah, NJ: Paulist Press, 2001.

O'Connor, Flannery. "The Enduring Chill." *The Complete Stories.* New York: Farrar, Straus and Giroux, 1971. 357–82.

—. "The Enduring Chill." *Harper's Bazaar,* July 1958: 44–45, 94, 96, 100–02, 108.

—. *The Habit of Being,* edited by Sally Fitzgerald. New York: Farrar, Straus and Giroux, 1979.

Parker, James N., and Philip M. Parker, eds. *Brucellosis: A Medical Dictionary, Bibliography, and Annotated Research Guide to Internet References.* San Diego: ICON Group International, 2004.

Parker, James N., and Philip M. Parker, eds. *The Official Patient's Sourcebook on Brucellosis*. San Diego: ICON Group International, 2002.

Poe, Edgar Allan. "A Descent Into the Maelström." *Poetry and Tales*. New York: Library of America, 1984. 432–48.

Spivey, Ted. *Flannery O'Connor: The Woman, the Thinker, the Visionary*. Macon, GA: Mercer University Press, 1995.

Whitt, Margaret Earley. *Understanding Flannery O'Connor*. Columbia: University of South Carolina Press, 1995.

Wood, Ralph C. *Flannery O'Connor and the Christ-Haunted South*. Grand Rapids, MI: William B. Eerdmans, 2004.

CHAPTER THREE

YEARS OF DISCRETION: CLYDE EDGERTON ON OLD AGE

JAN NORDBY GRETLUND

"It's a free country—unless you're old and in the way."
—Clyde Edgerton, *Lunch at the Piccadilly*.[1]

According to the US Census Bureau about 35.9 million Americans were older than sixty-five in the year 2003. The number is supposed to double by 2030. The figure for 2014 is close to forty million. Of the sixty-five year old about thirteen million live in the South, and it is a number that increases rapidly every year. In Clyde Edgerton's North Carolina almost 30 percent of people above sixty-five live alone, 36 percent if we focus on the women. Only 1.5 percent were older than eighty-five in the region, but that figure has grown by 50 percent in ten years. In the South 17 percent of those older than eighty-five live in nursing homes, this is, however, one number which is decreasing.[2] In order to illustrate the lingering southern concept of time, or the past in the present, Clyde Edgerton created Hansen County, North Carolina, which is the setting of much of his fiction, and his topics are often the extended family and their relationships. This is not just to illustrate a small town social comedy, it is also a postmodern interrogation into serious existential issues such as living, aging, and dying.

During my first interview with Clyde Edgerton, which was at Millsaps College, in Jackson, MS. in March, 1996, he told me:

---

[1] Clyde Edgerton, *Lunch at the Picadilly: A Novel* (Chapel Hill, NC: Algonquin Books, 2003), 197.

[2] "Age and Sex Composition in the United States: 2012." United States Census Bureau. http://www.census.gov/population/age/data/2012comp.html

> My parents' experience had been exactly that of their grandparents, in many ways. The physical environment and social norms, cultural and religious norms, were what had happened to their parents and grandparents and great-grandparents. What happened to me? It turned out I went away to college, to Chapel Hill, and the resulting gap is in many ways what is interesting to me."[3]

In Clyde Edgerton's eleven novels, from *Raney* (1985) to *The Night Train* (2011), age and aging, and what we do with, and to, old people, are primary topics. There is an abundance of characters, many are old, some are dead, but still operating fully in the minds of the living. Many of the characters are also narrators and they tell us about their families and communities and often the history of *all* they remember, including ancestors long dead.

Edgerton describes old age as an extended period of losses: the loss of memory, the loss of skills, the loss of mobility, the loss of respect, the loss of dignity, the loss of manners, the loss of quality in living, the loss of influence (even on your immediate family), the loss of healthy food, the loss of privacy, the loss of control of your finances, the loss of personal hygiene, the loss of the ability to keep clean your much reduced living space, and the loss of the self through the interference of strangers. These include: nursing staff, television personalities, evangelists, and at times "forgotten" friends and probable and possible members of the family.

What is gained in old age is equally dismal; in the reduced life of old age you are likely to become sentimental, stingy, suspicious, and forced to eat food you do not like, such as fast food. On the other hand, enunciating "I know you will love it," old people will, maybe in self-defense or as pay-back, force long forgotten courses, such as a dish of fried okra, on young people.[4] Time is a presence in abundance, Edgerton describes it as "a very long hallway full of thick fog" with "a very, very dull glow at the end of the hall."[5] As Aunt Lil experiences it, time is "the strangest thing. It pulls up into a little bunch and just sits there, not even spread out anymore …. all of it gets wrapped up in a little bunch that seems about a year or two old, and it is right there behind you."[6] Even though they are aware that they are running out of time, some old people remain vain and are

---

[3] Jan Nordby Gretlund, Personal interview with Clyde Edgerton (Millsaps, 26 March, 1996).

[4] Clyde Edgerton, *Raney: A Novel* (Chapel Hill, NC: Algonquin Books, 1985), 73-75.

[5] Edgerton, *Lunch at the Picadilly*, 226-27.

[6] Ibid., 194-95.

increasingly concerned about their personal appearance, "what if you died in just your underwear," Pearl says, trying to convince Mattie, her younger sister of seventy-eight, to wear pajamas. [7]

The elderly may feel so lonely and isolated that they talk to themselves all the time and in extreme cases even teach themselves ventriloquism in order to be able to talk with somebody, anybody. Mrs. Albright, in *The Bible Salesman*, "throws her voice" so all her cats have individualized voices; and they have Biblical names. At one point the cat named Moses says, "Let my people go!" and Judas, another cat, says, "If I had a gun, I'd shoot myself."[8] The old are bored, and preoccupied with their "final days"; as defensive measures, Edgerton's old people are in denial of their physical *dis*abilities, they criticize the present, insist on embalming the memory of their early years, and, while trying to cut their toenails, they take comfort in *Jesus*.[9] Though in Mattie Rigsbee's opinion, it is a problem with Jesus that "it wadn't his way to come in and keep you company. You couldn't cook for him."[10]

The observation most often expressed among Edgerton's aging characters is "I'm gettin' so I can't remember nothing no more." What happens too often is that somebody goes into a big store and realizes she has forgotten what she came in for.[11] If they are in the right store, some of the old women are tight-fisted, even parsimonious, shoppers, such as Mattie in *Killer Diller.* In the manner of many old people she tells stories that include too many *irrelevant details*, so the stories become surprisingly and insufferably long for young people, who have increasingly shorter attention spans, but Mattie does get to the point of her story. Eventually she tries to explain her shopping experience to Wesley, a young man:

> "I went in Revco yesterday to get some corn pads," says Mattie. "You know you used to could get twelve for thirty-nine cents. Did you know that?"…."this was a box of nine for $1.44, marked down from $1.99. But the saleslady was some foreigner and I was thinking so hard about *her* I didn't notice until I got home that she had charged me $1.99. If I hadn't

---

[7] Clyde Edgerton, *Walking across Egypt: A Novel* (Chapel Hill, NC: Algonquin Books, 1987), 22-23.

[8] Clyde Edgerton, *The Bible Salesman: A Novel* (New York: Little, Brown and Company, 2008), 36-37.

[9] Toenail passages: Clyde Edgerton, *Killer Diller: A Novel* (Chapel Hill, NC: Algonquin, 1991), 83; Clyde Edgerton, *Where Trouble Sleeps: A Novel* (Chapel Hill, NC: Algonquin Books, 1997), 126-27; corn passages: Edgerton, *Walking across Egypt*, 1.

[10] Edgerton, *Walking across Egypt*, 76.

[11] Edgerton, *Killer Diller*, 84.

> needed one so bad I would have taken them back. Well, they were just the right size for this bad corn I got, so last night I got one out to put on…. Anyway, about the time I got ready to stick it on the corn, for some reason I had to get up to do something, and I thought to myself, I'll finish this in a minute. Well, when I got back to the couch I couldn't find the pad…. Couldn't find it nowhere. Finally I decide I'm going to have to get another one out of the package….Well, I want you to know that while I'm pulling the backing off the second one I feel something stuck to the heel of my hand and bless pat there it was—the lost one…. So—I saved it. That one. Used the other one. I'm not about to throw away a—what would that be?—a twenty-cent corn pad."[12]

A feared result of aging is, of course, a loss of memory, and the result is confusion, even in doing something that you have done for many years, such as driving a car or for that matter wiping the toilet seat; if you do it using Listerine rather than alcohol, it will kill the germs, but it becomes sticky.[13] The simple forgetting of what you are doing, while you are trying to do it, is a sign of aging. The old Blaine sisters, Miss Bea and Miss Mae, who run the family store, are important characters in *Where Trouble Sleeps*. (Trouble is a dog that sleeps inside or outside in accordance with his weather expectations. People in town know that Trouble is always right.) The sisters cannot catch their chickens anymore, so they sneak up on them from behind, and shoot their heads off with their double-barreled 12-gauge shotgun. They communicate this important part of the Listre community culture to a young boy. "Don't you ever leave your mama and daddy. Do you hear me?" "Yes ma'am." "Now, do you want to learn how to shoot a chicken?" "Yes ma'am, I think so."[14] The sisters are always snapping at each other, always discussing important topics such as on which road did somebody live and who was the cousin of somebody's half-brother. Always fussing, always worried about what the other one is thinking, never wanting to be apart, but really needing to be.[15] Clyde Edgerton told me about his early youth with old people:

> As I grew up, my mother's favorite sisters were all in their early forties or late thirties when I was born, the three of them. So I am growing up, in many ways, with the undivided attention of these three women with one child. This was the norm for me. I heard a lot of their talking, I heard their language, and certainly felt their values, which in many ways were

---

[12] Ibid., 86-87.
[13] Edgerton, *Walking across Egypt*, 40
[14] Edgerton, *Where Trouble Sleeps*, 145.
[15] Ibid., 46.

somewhat different. So there was a kind of attention on *me*. Then came 'the gap' for me, when I left home and then came back and could see that I could still get along with them, visit with them, be with them, and talk to them. Some of that helped me write. Most of the absorption of stories was unconscious as I grew up. Most of the time the origin of the fiction would be little stories told about somebody else, on occasion I would make one up. A good amount of talk in the first several novels, especially, grew out of family stories, family talk.[16]

The Blaine Sisters with their expert knowledge of shotguns were chosen by Clyde Edgerton, as he told me, to revenge the grandmother, who was killed by the Misfit in Flannery O'Connor's short story "A Good Man is Hard to Find" (1955). The sisters find that a stranger, locally called "the gypsy man," is busy robbing their store. Miss Bea, one of the sisters, stops Mr. Jones, as he calls himself, with her shotgun:

> Jack Umstead [his real name] looked over his shoulder with calmness, an assurance that all would be well. He was, however, not expecting to be looking up the double barrels of a 12-gauge shotgun .... The no-count looked at her. 'Don't get no ideas,' she said. She made a little push motion with her gun. 'I'll shoot a hole in you big enough to stick my arm through.'"[17]

And when the intruder tries to charge at her, she shoots, one barrel at a time. "As he lay on the ground, still, the blood and hair let go little whiffs of smoke."[18]

> *Gretlund* Why do *you* want to kill off Jack Umstead, the 'gypsy man,' so badly? His not having a family, or any responsibility, hardly seems enough of a justification. He *is* killed off by the author, isn't he?
> *Edgerton* You are discovering secrets that should not be told. This was part of a short story that was written before the novel. It was named for Roy Acuff's "The Great Speckled Bird." It was a consequence of Flannery O'Connor killing off the old lady. I wanted to even that up. I wanted the old lady to kill off a bad man, a Misfit. So I evened up that score and felt good about it, and as I was writing the novel, it came to me that it would be a nice ending; it is no more complicated than that.[19]

---

[16] Gretlund 1996.
[17] Edgerton, *Where Trouble Sleeps*, 239-40.
[18] Ibid.
[19] Jan Nordby Gretlund, Personal interview with Clyde Edgerton (Wilmington, 29 September, 2010).

A popular story about the Blaine Sisters has one of them upstairs, half in and half out of the tub, she couldn't remember if she was getting *in* or *out* of the tub. So she calls out for her sister, but *she* is slow in getting there. She was stuck on the stairs, unable to remember whether she was going up or down. This story is told by a man who told it so often that he began to forget the story itself and once had to stop in the middle of telling it; which then became "a brand new story he told for a while – the story about forgetting the story."[20] The sisters' beginning senility is inherited, their mother lived with them for four years after their father died, fully convinced that her husband was still alive and always in some other room in the house. One of the sisters confesses, "It got to be real easy not to tell her he'd died."[21]

The worst kind of forgetfulness for anybody is, of course, when you cannot recognize your own kin. Lizzy Swanson's grandson, in *Trouble*, who lives in Tennessee and has not seen his grandmother in over twenty years, comes to visit with her, announcing "I'm David your grandson." Mrs. Swanson asks the young man to come in and have some cookies, and they sit down and she says "Now who'd you say you were?"… "*David* your grandson. You remember your daughter Betty, don't you?" …. "Yes, I remember Betty."… "Well, I am Betty's *son* and that makes me your *grandson.*" Mrs. Swanson leaned across the table looked him in the eye, and said: "That is too deep for me."[22] This is a story Edgerton used again in *Lunch at the Piccadilly*;[23] it is, of course, a passage that mocks forgetfulness, or perhaps mocks the postmodern theater. As it reads, it might well have been a passage from Harold Pinter's *The Dumb Waiter* (1957) or from Samuel Beckett's *Endgame*, (1958) plays that deliberately underestimate and mock old people, in order to bring out the reduction of everybody. *Lunch* has a similar 'postmodern' dialogue set in the Piccadilly restaurant of the title of the novel: because she is old, a young man carries Aunt Lil's tray ahead to the table. But Aunt Lil stops before she reaches the table and says: "'Have we eaten yet? Or are we about to eat.' 'I already got my food?' 'Yes ma'am. It's over there on the table.' 'What did I get?' 'Fried chicken.' 'Oh.' She starts walking again. 'I'm not surprised.'"[24] On the other hand, food is something that many elderly focus on, maybe for lack of better conversation topics. Mattie will tell you what she had for lunch yesterday. Her selective memory can bring up every item, separately:

---

[20] Edgerton, *Where Trouble Sleeps*, 42.
[21] Ibid., 49.
[22] Ibid., 42-43.
[23] Edgerton, *Lunch at the Picadilly*, 192.
[24] Ibid., 151-52.

"Fish, the fish sauce, peas, which was mushy, though not as mushy as they have been, carrots, slaw." What is more surprising perhaps is that she remembers every item on the plates of the two people she was with. Most surprising is perhaps, that she also remembers in detail what the people at the next table had.[25] Maybe we all have such observant family members?

Clyde Edgerton's *Lunch at the Piccadilly* is one of the best novels ever with its topic solidly planted in a nursing home for the elderly. It is called Rosehaven Convalescence Home. Even if parts of the South are less depersonalized than so many other places, even today, the novel demonstrates clearly what we do with old people, when we stack "the local wrecks of local women along the grim halls of local nursing homes,"[26] where they become "invisible people" without separate identities. Old people, mouths open, looking for somebody to come in; some of them will get up and follow you down the hall, hoping they know you. Living in a nursing home is difficult and worrying, not only because of the fear of death, but also because it is expensive to be there. The elderly are often exploited financially. Edgerton suggests that we ask the money-making churches to take responsibility for the elderly—especially when their home health care runs out—by joining with the money-making nursing homes. The elderly think there is too much business, Mrs. Satterwhite wonders: "What's dot-com? They keep saying it on television,"[27] and also that there are too many companies, she says, trying to take over the world, "like Hitler."[28] The companies interfere with the old people's lives by sending them bills, written in light blue letters, in a font that nobody can read without a magnifying glass; the letters arrive in their own return envelopes, which nobody can open, not to mention *fold* to return.

> *Gretlund* Your notion of setting up nursing homes in the generally vacant churches is, of course, ingenious. What could be more natural for good Christians than to help needy old people, so nursing homes and churches would be synonymous? How was your idea of creating 'Nurches' received? Has it been picked up yet by any of the TV evangelists?
> *Edgerton* Not yet! The play [based on *Lunch at the Piccadilly*] brings it to life. The play and the musical, in particular, differ somewhat from the novel.[29]

---

[25] Edgerton, *Killer Diller*, 87.
[26] Edgerton, *Lunch at the Picadilly*, 190.
[27] Ibid., 186.
[28] Ibid., 164.
[29] Gretlund 2010.

Would it not be a great Christian idea to create nurches with space and money enough for old people to end their lives comfortably and with dignity, purpose, and humor, in space provided by the nurches. "Why should churches and nursing homes not be interchangeable?"[30] Why should they not want to ease suffering among the wrinkled? Who needs to hear about the Last Supper when they are in need of the First Breakfast?[31]

This is, of course, severe social criticism by Edgerton, also of the two institutions named. In many countries elderly people are *respected*, one "inmate" suggests, but not "among us proud-to-be-all-powerful Americans."[32] As it is, we might as well go back a hundred thousand years, one of the old guys declares, when "we lef' old people under a tree, or et … ate them so we could go on and … take care of the chi'ren …."[33] The least you could ask of the Nurches of America is that they "diminish the force of fast food," now that they have already "completely ruint corn bread."[34] Some of the elderly "inmates" are fat from shame and boredom, their memory would benefit from some properly cooked traditional food. It would be an improvement if old people did not have to steal food from restaurants such as the Golden Corral or Morrison's; which is often difficult anyway, as hardly anybody from the nursing homes drives a car anymore.

> *Gretlund* In *Lunch at the Piccadilly* (2003) there is a good deal of serious criticism of how we treat the elderly. From page one it is criticism aimed at Medicare and Medicaid. Are the homes for the elderly and the daycare centers nothing but business and simple exploitation?
> *Edgerton* In any endeavor in which we try to care for those who are less fortunate than we are, there are mixed consequences. And of course, as always the room in the human heart which embraces greed goes to work. There clearly are people who are taking advantage of precious human lives. There are also genuine efforts in old age homes, for sure, and in nursing homes, many times by conservative fundamentalist Christians. As a person who is *not* a fundamentalist it is easy to jump on and satirize, but there is also a constancy in care for the poor among some of these religious people which makes you pause and think about how humane they are.
> I was not trying so much to make a statement, but I did jump on Medicare, for what happened to me, leading up to this book, were, of course, three years with an elderly aunt who had no one to care for her, except for me. So I got to see the inside of all this, I had to do the Medicare forms, the kind of things that any bureaucracy puts you through, and something to be

[30] Edgerton *Lunch at the Picadilly*, 62.
[31] Ibid., 64.
[32] Ibid., 163.
[33] Ibid., 239.
[34] Ibid., 202.

> satirized. I remember having fun with that and not knowing where to put it …. I have a feeling, for what it is worth, that in two hundred years when we look at ourselves as a society, we will see our treatment of older people, as something that we had turned a blind eye towards.[35]

It is in a description of Aunt Lil that Edgerton writes his most moving portrait of old age. She is just falling asleep in her room at Rosehaven and wants to sleep, to the extent the floodlight, placed right outside her window, will permit it. She has a photo of her business-school friends on the wall. It seems to her, in her half-awake state, that one after the other the old friends grow and step carefully out of the photograph and into her room.

> She wants badly to remember their names, but she can't. In her room, they make themselves at home, looking around, separating the blinds and looking out the window, helping themselves to Tootsie Rolls. Lil realizes that if she stays very still, they will not know she is there and she will not embarrass herself by speaking to them without remembering their names.[36]

Aunt Sarah, Aunt Lil's sister, ("Aunt Sarah, who once said that if she'd known she was going to live as long as she did, she'd have bought a new mattress") maintained that "stopping driving was the worst thing that she'd ever been through," and the statement came from a woman who had been through some bad times: she had lost her husband, her daughter had had a bad divorce, and she had watched her dog Skippy get run over.[37] There is no doubt that, particularly in the American society, a good deal of your identity goes when you cannot or are *not allowed* to drive anymore. This is not just the loss of another skill, which is bad enough, but the loss of your mobility. The right to roam all over without restriction or supervision is deeply anchored in the American identity. It is Carl Turnage's unpleasant task to tell his Aunt Lil that "today will probably be the last time you will drive a car," and he has a hard time trying to say just that.

Aunt Lil is dressed to go to town in her golden slippers, slacks, Hawaiian shirt, striped jacket, and "makeup that stops along her jaw like the border of a country,"[38] and she has to bring her walker. She does not recognize her car, it's been washed. But she is determined to show that she can drive as well as anybody, and she trusts that her hands and feet will

---

[35] Gretlund 2010.
[36] Edgerton, *Lunch at the Picadilly*, 220
[37] Ibid., 6-7.
[38] Ibid., 5.

remember what to do, just as they would remember riding a bicycle. Going for "the exit" she goes down a straight ramp and runs against the curb, several times. She asks her nephew "Am I driving?" which Carl confirms, and they stop at the bottom of the ramp. She believes that she was too low in the seat and needs more padding under her. The nephew does not think this is her basic problem. He asks her to put the car in park, and he walks around the car determined to tell her, as gently as possible, that she has to give up driving, only to see the car rolling slowly away and her golden slippers hanging out the door. With her feet sticking out Aunt Lil still drives, but she cannot understand where her nephew went. He sees her eyes slightly above the steering wheel just before he runs his head straight into a column. In spite of his head injury, Carl manages to get into the car and pull the break. Aunt Lil's first words to him are, "Where did you go?" "You drove off without me, Aunt Lil." "Why?" she asks.[39] He feels sorry for her, and knowing she dreads any comment on her driving, he decides to postpone the necessary conversation until they get back to Rosehaven. It is a powerful scene that brings out the helplessness of both of them in the face of advancing age, the loss of a necessary skill, and the loss of an important part of her identity. Aunt Lil does not want "to beg about anything," she still thinks the time will come when she can *drive* back to her apartment and "take up where she left off." But she realizes that "giving up driving would be the first mile of a highway that leads to a permanent spot" in the nursing home.[40]

On the other hand in the later Edgerton novel *The Bible Salesman*, Mrs. Sarah Finley, who is ninety-one now, and looks ninety-eight, still drives. Even though she claims, "I didn't kiss my husband afore we was married and I didn't kiss him after," she gave birth to eleven children, besides two she lost. She is another of Edgerton's admirable, tough, stoic women; Mrs. Finley fell in the garden one day and lay in the corn rows, possibly with a stroke, and could not get up, so until she was found she weeded as far as she could reach.[41] Some old people, such as the Bissetts, portrayed in *The Night Train*, have the advantage of living with their spouse until ripe old age. The Bissetts are now shut-ins and dependent on the delivery of food, etc. Mrs. Bissett is a small woman who talks "ninety miles an hour," whereas Mr. Bissett just sits and listens. They were born during the Civil War, she is ninety-nine and he is a hundred, but still driving his '39 Ford. They have been married for seventy-five years, but she still calls him "sweetheart." A young man is impressed with Mrs.

[39] Ibid., 16.
[40] Ibid., 174.
[41] Edgerton, *The Bible Salesman*, 121-22.

Bissett's use of a term of endearment at her age, but his uncle explains that she may be calling her husband "sweetheart," because she no longer remembers her groom's given name.[42]

Old people often wish for extensive families and hope, sometimes insist, their children give them many grandchildren. Mattie Rigsbee of the novels *Walking across Egypt* and *Killer* does not want to die without grandchildren. She is desperate, her son of forty-three and her daughter of thirty-eight never date the same people for more than a year or so, and every week the chances for grandchildren grow slimmer. "If they didn't hurry it would be too late to have children," Mattie believes. "It was her duty to remind them. That was a main reason mothers existed. To remind. And now chances looked slim."[43] She tries to talk with Elaine, but her daughter's answer is always something about career goals and equal opportunity. Once the would-be grandmother even insists that she herself is getting married and plans to rent, or adopt, so she can have 'grandchildren' of her own. And she insists on talking on the phone with Winston Sullivan, her daughter's friend, a conversation that begins: "Do you have any intention of marrying Elaine?" and ends in an even more disturbing exchange:

> "How's your sperm?" "Beg your pardon?" "I said how's your sperm; how old are you?" "I'm forty-seven. I hadn't checked my sper—" "Your sperm starts getting weak when you pass forty-four." Mattie says good-bye to Winston, who is now greatly uncomfortable. To her daughter, Mattie says: "He sounds like a nice young man but it's time he was going home. Or getting married. His sperm is getting tired."[44]

Mattie finally does become a grandmother when she accepts to become the guardian of Wesley Benfield, a juvenile delinquent of sixteen, who is released to her and becomes her much wanted 'grandson.' Mattie never has any reason to regret taking on the responsibility.

Whereas they do not see any problems with their own, often unexpected and unconventional, actions old people *will* criticize the present and deplore the loss of the past. Mattie Rigsbee, whom you know by now, and Grove McCord, of Edgerton's novel *In Memory of Junior*, *are* the past in the present. Grove says repeatedly "you're history longer than you're fact," but people seem to ignore that.[45] Both are worried about

---

[42] Edgerton, *The Night Train*, 105-106.
[43] Edgerton, *Walking across Egypt*, 50-51, 76.
[44] Ibid., 209-11.
[45] Edgerton, *In Memory of Junior*, 66, 142.

the decline of the values of the past, now we no longer have marriage, generations, manners, decent speech, courtesy, and faith. Like other old people they are convinced "that courteousness had started on the way out with television and integration and a man on the moon," Mattie cannot pinpoint the exact connections or what could be done about it. Yet she and Grove both know that these are the reasons for the great decline of courtesy and the bad manners of today's children—even in church. And they *know* that "the weather had been affected by those people landing on the moon"[46]—or, as Grove sees it: "When they started messing with the moon, and people's habits and manners and likes and *personal* dislikes and *personal* preferences, and started mixing the races, they went too far."[47]

In Memory of Junior is focused on age and on race. Grove McCord fears his final time on earth and plans his own burial. He has lived most of his life in Arkansas, but now that he expects to die, and wants to; he is "coming home" to be buried with his family in North Carolina. He prefers to lay out his grave himself and to do it now, rather than to face the frightening prospect of years in a nursing home or in a hospital. His daughter thinks he is getting senile, which she will state clearly although her father is present, because she thinks he cannot hear; but Grove claims he "can hear a cricket fart in a fast-moving train."[48] Much more than a reduction of his mental capacity, he fears the physical deterioration as a degrading, unpleasant, and sad end to life:

> "I ain't gone get hooked up on no tubes and all that with them foreign juices flowing in my body from no telling where, full of germs, little blip blip machines going off all over the place, people I don't know from Adam coming in sticking their finger up my ass and all that. You think I'm gone let myself in for that? Why hell no, why should I get stuck dying for eight or ten years."[49]

He then begins to dig his grave, and one midnight as he is kneeling next to his box-like coffin, Grove solemnly declares: "Papa, papa. I'm coming to join you. It's the only thing left to do. I'm shitting down my leg every few days now. People have to clean me up. There ain't nowhere else to go." Fully convinced that "dying is a part of living," as Pearl maintains,[50] Grove

---

[46] Edgerton, *Walking across Egypt*, 85, 87-88.
[47] Edgerton, *In Memory of Junior*, 72.
[48] Ibid., 131.
[49] Ibid., 128.
[50] Edgerton, *Walking across Egypt*, 43.

gets in the box, puts the lid on from inside, and falls asleep. He has hired a young black man, who thinks the old guy "has some stuck valves," to come and fill in the grave in the morning.[51] If you want to know more, read the novel.

Edgerton's 2011 novel *The Night Train* is mainly about race, music, and integration in North Carolina in the year 1963. One of the considerations for the old white people in town is that they hope to have *white* help when they get to be too old to manage on their own, but unless they are well off, they have to manage with "colored women from across the tracks."[52]

The novel *Redeye*, set in the American West in 1891, brings us from would-be grandmothers in the present to ancient mummies from the past, *and* throws in one silent grandmother. The embalmed past is being unearthed, because there is money in displaying desert-dried native mummies. Mr. Blankenship explains, "Do you realize what your average man from New York City or Philadelphia would pay to see a mummy that's been around since before the Egyptian pharaohs? …. And we'd be doing the world of culture and colleges and universities a great favor."[53] They apply electricity to a mummy to bring her back to life with "a divine spark" and they claim she sat up, talked, and ate some oatmeal, but the electricity burnt a hole in her chest and she died again. When they find an almost perfect mummified baby, who looks "almost alive except she was staring out of little dark holes," they decide to make some money by exhibiting the mummies.[54]

They learn about embalming and use Glo-Tex on Grandmother Copeland for the pallor; she is alive and in a roller-chair, but has to be in the display. They need her to have a complete family of mummies. "Cleopatra," the woman mummy they found, is dressed up as a man, and grandmother Copeland, who never speaks, refuses to let go of the baby mummy, and hollers when they try to take it from her arms, believing it to be one of four babies she lost long ago. She is appointed mama mummy and tries to nurse the baby mummy. Cobb Pittman, the owner of Redeye, the dog of the title, is outraged and speaks to the grandmother: "What the hell do you think you're doing?" …"That baby is a mummy. I ought to sic my dog on your baby." She looked at the baby. "You're going to hell when you die. And your baby, too." She looked back at me and smiled.

---

[51] Edgerton, *In Memory of Junior*, 153-56
[52] Edgerton, *The Night Train*, 147, 168.
[53] Clyde Edgerton, *Redeye: A Western* (Chapel Hill, NC: Algonquin Books, 1995), 153.
[54] Ibid., 166-67.

"Kiss yo mammy's ass." After that Pittman got up and left her alone; he figured all along she could talk. His general complaint is that "used to there weren't no women or babies much out here. Now it's grandmas and mummies."[55]

What does the young generation, even in Hansen County, North Carolina, care about the old and the dying, and/or their grandparents, if they only get to know them as somebody locked up in a nursing institution. Edgerton's view of old age and the process of aging is reflected in his elderly characters, who, on one hand, range from the very active, almost heroic, such as Mattie Rigsbee and Grove McCord, who certainly are not reduced, physically or mentally, to the much frailer Blaine Sisters and Aunt Lil, women who are still active but suffer from the loss of memory, which means that many challenges cannot be met. In this way aging is highly individualized in Edgerton's fictional universe, but it is suggested that time will eventually set back even the most spirited of us. Only people who die early enough are likely to escape the losses and reduction of old age.

Works Cited

"Age and Sex Composition in the United States: 2012." United States Census Bureau. http://www.census.gov/population/age/data/2012comp.html

Edgerton, Clyde. *In Memory of Junior: A Novel.* Chapel Hill, NC: Algonquin Books, 1992.

—. *The Bible Salesman: A Novel.* New York: Little, Brown and Company, 2008.

—. *Killer Diller A Novel.* Chapel Hill, NC: Algonquin, 1991.

—. *Lunch at the Piccadilly: A Novel.* Chapel Hill, NC: Algonquin Books, 2003.

—. *The Night Train.* New York: Little, Brown and Company, 2011.

—. *Raney: A Novel.* Chapel Hill, NC: Algonquin Books, 1985.

—. *Redeye: A Western.* Chapel Hill, NC: Algonquin Books, 1995.

—. *Where Trouble Sleeps: A Novel.* Chapel Hill, NC: Algonquin Books, 1997.

—. *Walking across Egypt: A Novel.* Chapel Hill, NC: Algonquin Books, 1987.

Gretlund, Jan Nordby, Personal interview with Clyde Edgerton. Millsaps, March 26, 1996.

---

[55] Ibid., 206-207.

—. Personal interview with Clyde Edgerton. Wilmington, September 29, 2010.

Grimshaw, Jr., James A. "Clyde Edgerton: Death and Dying," *Southern Writers at Century's End*, edited by Jeffrey J. Folks and James Perkins, 238-46. Lexington: The University Press of Kentucky, 1997.

Romine, Scott. "Epilogue: Whence the Community? Some Thoughts on Contemporary Southern Literature," *The Narrative Forms of Southern Community*, 196-211.Baton Rouge: Louisiana State University Press, 1999.

PART II:

PSYCHOLOGICAL DISORDERS

CHAPTER FOUR

SOUTHERN EVIL, SOUTHERN VIOLENCE: GOTHIC RESIDUES IN THE WORKS OF WILLIAM GAY, BARRY HANNAH, AND CORMAC MCCARTHY

THOMAS ÆRVOLD BJERRE

I

Southern literature has a long tradition of depicting violence and depravity. Ever since the haunting Gothicism of Edgar Allan Poe, southern writers have tapped into the eerie tradition and used it to depict an atmosphere of the uncanny—as seen in the works of William Faulkner, Flannery O'Connor, Truman Capote, and Eudora Welty. Today's many southern writers still draw on elements of the Gothic to depict a world of violence and anxiety. As Jerrold E. Hogle asserts, addressing the Gothic in general, since the eighteenth century, Gothic fiction has enabled us to "address and disguise some of the most important desires, quandaries, and sources of anxiety, from the most internal and mental to the widely social and cultural…"[1] In an American context, Eric Savoy explains, the Gothic "embodies and gives voice to the dark nightmare that is the underside of 'the American Dream' …. It reveals the limitations of American faith in social and material progress." Savoy furthermore points out "the odd centrality of Gothic cultural production in the United States, where the past constantly inhabits the present, where progress generates an almost unbearable anxiety about its costs, and where an insatiable appetite for

[1] Jerrold E. Hogle, "Introduction," *The Cambridge Companion to Gothic Fiction*, ed. Jerrold E. Hogle (Cambridge: Cambridge University Press, 2002), 4.

spectacles of grotesque violence is part of the texture of everyday life."[2] An important part of the Gothic tradition is

> *prosopopoeia* or personification, by which abstract ideas (such as the burden of historical causes) are given a 'body' in the spectral figure of the ghost. It is also the strategy that enables the dead to rise, the ghostly voice to materialize out of nowhere, and objects to assume a menacing pseudo-life. It thus achieves the ultimate effects of the haunted, the uncanny, and the return of the repressed while placing these thoroughly in the depths of American life and the American psyche.[3]

Nowhere in the US is the Gothic more present than in the South, which Allison Graham describes as a "repository of national repressions… the benighted area 'down there' whose exposure to the light is unfailingly horrifying and thrilling."[4] Flannery O'Connor famously declared that the so-called "Southern school" of literature conjured up "an image of Gothic monstrosities and the idea of a preoccupation with everything deformed and grotesque."[5] Add to this Benjamin Fisher's definition of the literary Gothic as something that evokes "anxieties, fears, terrors, often in tandem with violence, brutality, rampant sexual impulses, and death,"[6] and it becomes clear how the tradition of the Southern Gothic plays into already established ideas about the South as an "ill" region. Charles Reagan Wilson notes how the "deadly climate that nurtured diseases" killed off early Jamestown settlers and later colonists in Lowcountry North Carolina, creating in turn an image of the South as "a death trap."[7]

This image coincided with what soon became the stereotype of the "Fighting South": a pathology of violence based on the "supposed proclivity

---

[2] Eric Savoy, "The Rise of the American Gothic," *The Cambridge Companion to Gothic Fiction*, ed. Jerrold E. Hogle (Cambridge: Cambridge University Press, 2002), 167.

[3] Ibid., 168.

[4] Allison Graham, "The South in Popular Culture," *A Companion to the Literature and Culture of the American South*, eds. Richard Gray and Owen Robinson (Malden, MA: Blackwell Publishing, 2007), 349.

[5] Flannery O'Connor, "The Fiction Writer & His Country," *Mystery and Manners: Occasional Prose*, eds. Sally and Robert Fitzgerald (1969; New York: Farrar, Straus & Giroux, 2000), 28.

[6] Benjamin F. Fisher IV, "Southern Gothic," *The New Encyclopedia of Southern Culture, vol. 9: Literature*, ed. M. Thomas Inge (Chapel Hill, NC: The University of North Carolina Press, 2008), 145.

[7] Charles Reagan Wilson, "Myth, Manners, and Memory," *The New Encyclopedia of Southern Culture, vol. 4: Myth, Manners, and Memory*, ed. Charles Reagan Wilson (Chapel Hill: The University of North Carolina Press, 2006), 1.

of" southerners "toward personal and societal violence."[8] Robert E. May notes how antebellum European and northern travelers reported "that the southern people enjoyed soldiering and resolved interpersonal disputes with violence to an unusual degree."[9] And the image of a violent South spans class boundaries. As Bertram Wyatt-Brown has shown, the duel is an example of how violence was "a part of the social order even in the upper ranks."[10] At the other end of the spectrum is the redneck stereotype, whose "essential characteristic," as John Shelton Reed explains, is "meanness." He "fights because he wants to *hurt* somebody, often somebody helpless." Reed argues that to a certain extent the violent redneck even became the dominant American view of the working-class white southern male, not least thanks to his regular appearance in popular culture.[11]

In the following, I will examine three contemporary practitioners of the Southern Gothic and the use of violence in their novels. The writers and their novels—William Gay's *The Long Home* (1999), Barry Hannah's *Yonder Stands You Orphan* (2001), and Cormac McCarthy's *No Country for Old Men* (2005)—all borrow various elements of the Gothic to support their bleak portrayals of the American South in which violence plays a crucial part. In these novels, the antagonists are violent men of seemingly pure evil, men driven by incredible blood-thirst who will stop at nothing to satisfy their deadly desires. Invoking the Gothic tradition, these villains take on the shape of ghosts or living dead, but apart from the obvious sensationalism provided by these killers, the writers use the villains symbolically in order to point out inherent problems in today's society and, more specifically, in the South.

Taken together, the three novels depict the American South as a region that has lost any sense of spirituality and instead has devoured itself in unscrupulous greed. The pessimistic portrayal of the New South echoes John Egerton's 1974 jeremiad *The Americanization of Dixie: The Southernization of America*, a book that, in Dwight Garner's words,

---

[8] Robert E. May, "Fighting South," "Myth, Manners, and Memory," *The New Encyclopedia of Southern Culture, vol. 4: Myth, Manners, and Memory*, ed. Charles Reagan Wilson (Chapel Hill: The University of North Carolina Press, 2006), 68.

[9] Ibid.

[10] Bertram Wyatt-Brown, *Honor and Violence in the Old South* (New York: Oxford University Press, 1986), 144-45.

[11] John Shelton Reed, *Southern Folk, Plain & Fancy: Native White Social Types* (Athens: The University of Georgia Press, 1986), 40.

criticized "how malled-up and hollow-souled the South was becoming."[12] It is a critique that most recently has been followed up by Tracy Thompson who states that "the South has been urbanized, suburbanized, strip-malled, and land-formed" almost beyond recognition.[13] The novels progress towards an increasingly negative worldview; I will begin in with the more positive of the three.

II

William Gay's debut novel *The Long Home* is a traditional tale of good versus evil set in a small Tennessee community in the 1950s. The heroes of the novel are the young carpenter Nathan and his friend, the old hermit William Tell Oliver. The evil villain is Dallas Hardin, a bootlegger and entrepreneur who has bribed and threatened the local top officials to silence, and who through a combination of physical violence and threats of more keeps the community cowed with fear:

> Short of killing him, how would you ensure the sanctity of your home, your family? Doors will burn, windows melt… locks blacken and lie unrecognizable among the ashes. When will he come, what will be the hour? …. He is a bearer of grudges, trifles drive him to limits an ordinary man only reads about.[14]

Hardin's evil is demonstrated in the opening pages when he secretly kills Nathan's father. Years later, when Nathan and Hardin's stepdaughter become romantically involved, the conflict between good and evil is inevitable. Dallas Hardin is obviously the personification of evil, a human being as worst-case scenario, and Gay imbues him with Gothic undertones: Like the devil reincarnated, Hardin appears in the community after an earthquake has opened a brimstone-smelling abyss in the ground. The locals feel uneasy after they have heard him talk about his origins, which display an extreme element of the Gothic: Hardin refers to himself as "a walkin dead man" because "he was born in a casket." His mother was

---

[12] Dwight Garner, "Crisscrossing a Region of Strip Malls and Ghosts," The New York Times, April 23, 2013. See John Egerton, *The Americanization of Dixie: The Southernization of America* (New York: Harper's Magazine Press, 1974).
[13] Tracy Thompson, *The New Mind of the South* (New York: Simon & Schuster, 2013), 235.
[14] William Gay, *The Long Home* (Denver, CO.: MacMurray & Beck, 1999), 48.

killed when pregnant, and during her funeral the congregation "heard a baby squallin [and Hardin] was down there in her clothes."[15]

The way Gay describes Hardin leaves no doubt as to his role in the novel:

> Over the years Hardin had taken on the lineaments of evil .... [His] vulpine face was leaner and more cunning than ever, the cold yellow eyes more reptilian. Or sharklike, perhaps, lifeless and blank save a perpetual look of avarice. And he went through life the way a shark feeds, taking into its belly anything that attracts its attention .... There was a gemlike core of malevolence beneath the sly grin, beneath the fabric of myth the years had clothed him in. In these myths he supplanted the devil, the tooth-and-claw monsters of childhood darkness.[16]

This paragraph reveals several interesting depictions of Hardin; not only is he compared to vicious-looking beasts, but evil is intrinsically linked to greed. And greed is what Hardin is meant to symbolize. Pitched against the young and idealistic carpenter hero, it becomes clear that the brutal and selfish Hardin represents greedy capitalism at its worst. His honky tonk preys on the weak community, and he uses violence to assert his power. The novel builds up the conflict between good and evil—Hardin is also referred to as "remorseless and implacable as an Old Testament God" and an "evil king"[17]—and in the classic tradition, the hero must resort to violence to overcome the villain. Old man William Tell Oliver steps in to prevent the young Nathan from becoming a killer. Oliver, who has a violent past, uses his wisdom actively and kills off Dallas Hardin.

In Gay's world then, violence does not necessarily equate evil. Furthermore, the apparent Gothic vision that is suggested by the depiction of Hardin is not carried through. The repressed evil that returns to haunt the community is successfully checked, and the dead Hardin is thrown back into the abyss from whence it is suggested he arrived. In Gay's world of good and evil, good ultimately triumphs through violence, or, to use pathological terms, violence can be said to have a healing potential. But the triumph does come with a price: after fulfilling his duty, Oliver retreats back to the wilderness from which he came. This retreat can both be seen as a continuous denunciation of civilized society, but there is also

---

[15] Ibid., 113.
[16] Ibid., 45-46.
[17] Ibid., 166, 174.

a touch of tragedy to the lone hero forced by his past burdens to live a life in solitude.[18]

III

Although Barry Hannah also unleashes evil upon a small community, his world is a bit more blurred than Gay's dichotomy of good and evil. Hannah's fiction features a wide array of killers, but the most intriguing is found in his last novel, *Yonder Stands Your Orphan*, in Man Mortimer, a charismatic Conway Twitty look-alike who is also a pedophile pimp and murderer.

Like Gay, Hannah employs aspects of the Gothic, but in a more playful, postmodern way. As one reviewer put it, the novel "crawls with the pulp of a cheap Gothic."[19] A decade before zombies experienced a popular rebirth with AMC's *The Walking Dead*[20] (which takes place in Georgia), Hannah used the image of the zombie to describe the decrepit state of the South. It is a region where casinos and pawnshops have ushered in a "Cash for Your Title civilization" and "pawnshop villages"[21] with "Quick cash, a lot of crack heads, a lot of people you didn't see before. Kind of dirty and needy folk in a new way …. they're depraved instantly if they don't hit the jackpot."[22] In the novel, the Mississippi Delta is now a rotten and degenerate place where the casino musicians, "although mistaken for the living by their audiences, *were* actually dead. Ghosts howling for egress from their tombs"[23]; a place where zombies

---

[18] For a discussion of how *The Long Home* employs themes from the American western, including the notion of what Richard Slotkin has called "regeneration through violence," see Thomas Ærvold Bjerre, "'Almost a Western': The Deep South as the Mythic West in William Gay's *The Long Home*, " *Moravian Journal of Literature and Film* 3, no. 1 (2011): 67-87.

[19] Shawn Badgley, "Readings," [review of *Yonder Stands Your Orphan*] *The Austin Chronicle*, Aug. 17, 2001.

[20] *The Walking Dead*, AMC, 2010-. It should be noted that the immensely popular TV series is based on the graphic adaptation by Robert Kirkman and Tony Moore from 2003, one that took place in Kentucky. In terms of Hannah's novel, the cover of the UK paperback version published by Atlantic Books (ISBN 1843540061) stresses the gothic setting and the zombie connotations. The image by Dave McKean depicts a pale hand reaching out through a hole in a locked door.

[21] Barry Hannah, *Yonder Stands Your Orphan* (New York: Atlantic Monthly Press, 2001), 117.

[22] Thomas Ærvold Bjerre, "Personal Interview with Barry Hannah," Athens, Ohio, May 11, 2001.

[23] Barry Hannah, *Yonder Stands Your Orphan*, 38-39

patronize "the bad restaurant" which "served food for the dead," and a place where zombies wait behind the counters of the countless pawnshops, "quite obviously dead and lead by someone beyond."[24] Hannah's use of zombie metaphors plays in to a well-established tradition of the living dead serving as a critique of "consumer capitalism."[25] and also points forward to Henry A. Giroux's analysis of contemporary American society in his book *Zombie Politics and Culture in the Age of Casino Capitalism.* Published ten years after Hannah's novel, Giroux's characterization of contemporary society is a more detailed echo of Hannah's Gothic vision:

> A casino capitalist zombie politics views competition as a form of social combat, celebrates war as an extension of politics, and legitimates a ruthless Social Darwinism in which particular individuals and groups are considered simply redundant, disposable—nothing more than human waste left to stew in their own misfortune—easy prey for the zombies who have a ravenous appetite for chaos and revel in apocalyptic visions filled with destruction, decay, abandoned houses, burned-out cars, gutted landscapes, and trashed gas stations.[26]

The fact that "casino capitalism" and its effects is a national epidemics only stresses the increasing lack of unique southern traits and the continuous homogenization of the South that Hannah seems to lament. This lament is partly rooted in a nostalgia that affects the characters in the novel. As Scott Romine has argued, *Yonder Stands Your Orphan* is dominated by "the nostalgia industry," which, because it "offers an implicit alternative history, a located might-have-been"[27] appeals to Hannah's characters who feel dispossessed in the New South.

Romine also discusses Hannah's use of zombie metaphors and argues that the novel depicts a degenerate culture of "empty consumption," in which people are "easy prey to the predators who command the economy of false gratification."[28] In this rotten South, Man Mortimer is king as

---

[24] Ibid., 175

[25] Stephanie Boluk and Wylie Lenz, "Introduction: Generation Z, the Age of Apocalypse," *Generation Zombie: Essays on the Living Dead in Modern Culture* (Jefferson, NC: McFarland & Company, 2011), 11.

[26] Henry A. Giroux, *Zombie Politics and Culture in the Age of Casino Capitalism* (New York: Peter Lang, 2011), 2.

[27] Scott Romine, "Orphans All: Reality Homesickness in *Yonder Stands Your Orphan*," *Perspectives on Barry Hannah*, ed. Martyn Bone (Jackson, MS: University Press of Mississippi, 2007), 168.

[28] Ibid., 166.

well as the predator that Romine mentions. Mortimer's reign of terror is brought on by the return of the repressed—a typical Gothic element: Six years previous to the action of the novel, Mortimer, who is horrified of commitment, was confronted by a woman and her six-year-old child, who claimed Mortimer as the father. When Mortimer denied, the woman shot her son, then herself. Shocked, Mortimer placed the bodies in the trunk of their car and drove it in the lake.[29] At the time the novel begins, a sinkhole drains the water in the lake, and the discovery of the bodies gets the story started. So in true Gothic fashion, the dead literally rise from the ground.

The dead bodies dumped in the bayou are an example of violence inherent in the landscape; a common theme in southern fiction, and one Gay also employed by having his villain seemingly appear from an abyss. In *Yonder Stands Your Orphan* nature has become a hiding place for past horrors; a mute witness to our history of evil. The Confederate and Union dead resting in the ground have been joined by other victims of horrible crimes:

> Scores of corpses rested below the lakes, oxbows, river ways and bayous of these parts, not counting the skeletons of Grant's infantry. The country was built to hide those dead by foul deed, it sucked at them. Back to the flood of 1927, lynchings, gun and knife duels were common stories here. Muddy water made a fine lost tomb."[30]

This points to Patricia Yaeger's assertion that "[b]odies of water are never simply sites for leisure or hauling cotton or crossing over but sites for recycling sadness."[31] These sites of sadness may explain or even encourage and spawn violent monsters like Man Mortimer. It is the resurfacing of the two dead bodies Mortimer buried in the bayou that unleashes his violent rampage. With their reappearance come guilt, responsibility, and a frightening display of the "insatiable appetite for spectacles of grotesque violence" that is one of the hallmarks of the Gothic.[32]

The reason for Mortimer's violent acts can be found in a deeply insecure masculinity. Robbed of his masculinity—he is stabbed in the crotch—Mortimer begins cutting people at random. Paradoxically, to

---

[29] Barry Hannah, *Yonder Stands Your Orphan*, 51.
[30] Ibid., 21-22.
[31] Patricia Yaeger, *Dirt and Desire: Reconstructing Southern Women's Writing 1930-1990* (Chicago: U of Chicago P, 2000), 13.
[32] Eric Savoy, "The Rise of the American Gothic," 167.

Mortimer, violence takes on a form of healing power. However, his obsession with knives and the consequent penetration of flesh clearly serve as a vicarious exercise in sexual intercourse. He stabs several men, slashes his girlfriend's thigh, and finally decapitates Pepper Farté, the old bait store owner.

Despite the psychological reasoning behind the violence, Mortimer is clearly a tool in what is basically a morality tale. He represents part of the greedy and rotten capitalist regime that is rearing its head in the New Casino South, which Hannah rages against. Mortimer's empire is built on the selling of flesh; much like the shark-like Dallas Hardin, Mortimer scavenges the casino exits for "ruined… women" he can "steer… to their salvation,"[33] and he also preys on the young orphan girls, hoping to get them in the porn videos he produces. By definition of his profession and morality (or lack thereof) Mortimer represents the modern world in all its insanity and he is clearly Hannah's epitome of all that is ill about the New South.

Against the evil embodied by Mortimer, Hannah's voice of reason is found in the grotesque preacher Egan, "a reformed biker, gambler and drug addict," who injects holy water directly in his vein with a hypodermic needle and who preaches against the casino, "this nearby hell, a factory of thievery and broken hearts." In a tirade turned directly against Mortimer, Egan

> preached about hollow and slick men and slot-machine hags with no souls. The leering zombies schooled to rob the poor and sad in the name of fun. Worse than the liquor were the glamour and baying of Mammonites, who turned the soul into nothing but the arithmetic of want."[34]

By comparing Mortimer with Mammon, the biblical demon symbolizing material wealth or greed, Hannah directly links Mortimer to the devil, another proof that he symbolizes the evil "disease" that has taken over the South.

Against Mortimer's violent rampage, the local sheriff turns out to be totally inept, and the burden falls on Raymond, the protagonist of the novel. He is already an unlikely hero, and, not surprisingly, he fails miserably in his confrontation with Mortimer. He is stabbed in the back and his role as hero is forever punctured. Instead, Mortimer meets his match when he is severely beaten up by the junk yard-owner Peden. The

---

[33] Barry Hannah, *Yonder Stands Your Orphan*, 10-11.

[34] Ibid., 11.

humiliating beating puts an end to his middle age, and he has now "graduated into old."[35]

Unlike Hannah's other males, Mortimer does not find peace within himself, and perhaps this is his punishment. Instead of gunning down the villain, Hannah lets him simmer in a perpetual state of male confusion. Because of his insistence on a violent hegemonic discourse, redemption for Mortimer is impossible. Ultimately, Mortimer is not killed off, but his former powers are stripped off him, and he ends up in jail, an emasculated echo of his previous self, reduced to a "thing that was hardly anything but a big head with a mass of hair on it."[36] His strain of terror and violence has left everyone full, and he is never redeemed. Because the narrative draws on our preconceived expectations of a traditional climax where good triumphs over evil the lack of a plain closure to the narrative seems all the more startling.

Unlike the more uplifting closure to Gay's novel, Hannah's ends on a note of indifferent resignation. Mortimer's reign of evil may have been stopped, but that does not mean that good won. As Hannah himself explains,

> I don't think that evil ever is truly punished. It has its own end. I have also noticed that the law… as much law as we have… often can't touch really the evil, and that evil itself is absorbed by a community and it lives with it. And it just sort of 'wears out' the evil.[37]

IV

This blurring of the lines between good and evil brings us to Cormac McCarthy whose fiction is the bleakest of the three. McCarthy's first three novels owe an obvious debt to the tradition of the Southern Gothic. They depict a depraved South of necrophilia and incest, and above all violence. McCarthy's fiction is steeped in violence, a result of his philosophy of life, as he explained in a much quoted interview with *The New York Times*: "There's no such thing as life without bloodshed… I think the notion that the species can be improved in some way, that everyone could live in harmony, is a really dangerous idea."[38] In *No*

---

[35] Ibid., 295.
[36] Ibid., 336.
[37] Robert L. Hall, "Motorcycles, Hamburgers, and Lines You Can't Forget: An Interview with Barry Hannah." *Southern Scribe* 2., no. 11 (November 2001), n.p.
[38] Richard B. Woodward, "Cormac McCarthy's Venomous Fiction," *The New York Times*, April 19, 1992, section 6, 28.

Country for Old Men, McCarthy plays out his bleak philosophy, this time in the form of a suspense thriller about drug trafficking that in a postmodern manner borrows from established genres such as crime fiction, pulp fiction, the western, as well as the Gothic.

The novel takes place in South-west Texas, and it is perhaps a stretch to consider it a southern novel, but I will do so nonetheless.[39] Like the Judge in his ultra-violent anti-western *Blood Meridian*, *No Country* features a cynical killer that is almost out of this world: the psychopath hitman Anton Chigurh. Chigurh is the epitome of an almost unearthly evil too large for any hero to defeat. His preferred weapon is an air-compressed cattle gun that leaves a hole in the victims but no bullet. He kills at least twelve people in the novel, and Sheriff Bell, whose county has not had an unsolved homicide in forty-one years[40], finds himself at a loss when confronted with the seemingly senseless evil behind the acts. "*Somewhere out there is a true and living prophet of destruction and I don't want to confront him. I know he's real. I have seen his work*."[41]

Like Gay and Hannah, McCarthy invokes traits of the Gothic in his depiction of the villain. "*He's a ghost. But he's out there*," Bell states in one of several references to Chigurh as a ghost.[42] Jim Welsh reads the novel partly as an allegory and considers Chigurh "too spooky, too otherworldly to be 'real.'"[43] Like Dallas Hardin in *The Long Home*, Chigurh is also compared more directly to the devil, and just as Hannah did, McCarthy compares his villain with Mammon,[44] a biblical demon symbolizing material wealth or greed. As Manuel Broncano puts it, "of all the demons that tempt mankind, Mammon will certainly prove to be the one that succeeds in bringing it to its perdition through greed."[45] And exactly material wealth and greed that form the base of the drug-

---

[39] The main character Sheriff Bell, described as a "redneck sheriff in a hick town. In a hick state" (157), is in many ways a typical Southern character, and apart from the obviously south-western landscape, the both gothic and grotesque traits of the novel lend it an unmistakable Southern flair.

[40] Cormac McCarthy, *No Country for Old Men* (New York: Alfred A. Knopf, 2005), 217.

[41] Ibid., 4. Italics in original.

[42] Ibid., 248, also 299.

[43] Jim Welsh, "Borderline Evil: The Dark Side of Byzantium in *No Country for Old Men*, Novel and Film," *No Country for Old Men: From Novel to Film*, eds. Lynnea Chapman King, Rick Wallach, and Jim Welsh (Lanham, MA: Scarecrow Press, 2009), 74.

[44] Ibid., 298.

[45] Manuel Broncano, *Religion in Cormac McCarthy's Fiction: Apocryphal Borderlands* (New York: Routledge, 2014), 116.

trafficking is the real evil in the novel. As Bell puts it, "If you were Satan and you were settin around tryin to think up somethin that would just bring the human race to its knees what you would probably come up with is narcotics."[46] While Chigurh leaves a physical trail of destruction, he is as much a symbol of the greed and carnage of our cynical age as he is a real person. Welsh sees him as "the very personification of the Antichrist …. Like Death itself, he is larger than life, not merely a stereotype, but an allegorical abstraction."[47]

It also bears mentioning that Llewelyn Moss, the character who appears to be a goodhearted anti-hero, is ultimately undone by his own weakness. When he stumbles upon a horrific scene of bodies from a shoot-out, he finds a suitcase full of money and decides to take it. As Broncano asserts, he is "tempted by the demon of greed—that is, Mammon—and falls into the trap that the devil has designed for him…"[48]

In this novel, the voice of reason comes from the world-weary Sheriff Bell, whose chapters of first-person narration serve as the moral center of the novel. One reviewer called the novel "a jeremiad against the depravity that lurks on the horizon, the anguish that burns the borderland of the Americas."[49] Clearly, *No Country* can be read as a morality tale, just like Gay's and Hannah's novels, but in McCarthy's case, the message comes too late. Bell's musings on good and evil are just that; musings. Because of the overwhelming display of evil, Bell realizes that he does not dare face the monster, and he eventually throws in the towel: "*Now I aim to quit and a good part of it is just knowin that I wont be called on to hunt this man. I reckon he's a man.*"[50] His decision mirrors his shameful desertion of his men during World War II, an act he has kept to himself for thirty-six years. In true Gothic fashion, his repression of the past comes back with a vengeance, and at the end of the novel, Bell is bitter and shameful, and the killer Chigurh is still on the loose.

Like Gay and Hannah, McCarthy also implies that the land itself may harbor the evil that is loose. "This country will kill you in a heartbeat," Bell asserts, and later ponders this idea: "*I still keep thinking maybe it is something about the country … this country has got a strange history and*

---

[46] Cormac McCarthy, *No Country for Old Men*, 218.

[47] Welsh, "Borderline Evil," 74. Manuel Broncano also refers to Chigurh as playing "the role of a true Antichrist." Broncano, *Religion*, 115.

[48] Broncano, *Religion*, 118.

[49] William J. Cobb, "On the Border of Evil," *Houston Chronicle*, July 15, 2005.

[50] Cormac McCarthy, *No Country for Old Men*, 283.

a damned bloody one too."[51] This is McCarthy's desolate vision, clearly the bleakest of the three novels discussed here.

What ties these three novels together is the seething criticism of a society succumbing to increasing greed and materialism. There is a hint of the old southern Agrarian ideology to be found here, for sure, a conservative clinging to an idealized past that serves as a resistance to progress, but Gay, Hannah, and McCarthy are much more explicit in their methods. By drawing on the Gothic tradition, they give the vices a murderous face, and by imbuing their killers with evil of Biblical proportions, the writers create extremely violent morality tales, where evil is always clearly defined and furthermore seems to seep out of the landscape.

Despite the clear dichotomy of the morality tale, the novels rarely succumb to sentimentalism. Even though Gay's novel employs a formulaic resolution to the conflict and ends on a note of optimism, there is still plenty of Gothic darkness to muddy the waters. And the futility of goodness in the face of evil that we find in Hannah and McCarthy turn their novels into desolate statements about the state of the contemporary South. In this way, the writers continue the exploration of the underside of the American dream, so central to the Gothic, and they are proof that the Southern Gothic is still alive and kicking, more bloody and violent than ever.

Works Cited

Badgley, Shawn. "Readings," [review of *Yonder Stands Your Orphan*] *The Austin Chronicle*, August. 17, 2001. http://www.chrontourage.com/gyrobase/Issue/review?oid=oid%3A 82641

Bjerre, Thomas Ærvold. "'Almost a Western': The Deep South as the Mythic West in William Gay's *The Long Home.* " *Moravian Journal of Literature and Film* 3, no. 1 (2011): 67-87.

—. "Personal Interview with Barry Hannah," Athens, Ohio, May 11, 2001.

Boluk, Stephanie and Wylie Lenz. "Introduction: Generation Z, the Age of Apocalypse." *Generation Zombie: Essays on the Living Dead in Modern Culture*, edited by Stephanie Boluk and Wylie Lenz, 1-17. Jefferson, NC: McFarland & Company, 2011.

Broncano, Manuel. *Religion in Cormac McCarthy's Fiction: Apocryphal Borderlands*. New York: Routledge, 2014.

[51] Ibid., 271, 284.

Cobb, William J. "On the Border of Evil." *Houston Chronicle*, July 15, 2005.
http://www.chron.com/disp/story.mpl/ae/books/reviews/3266816.html

Egerton, John. *The Americanization of Dixie: The Southernization of America*. New York: Harper's Magazine Press, 1974.

Fisher IV, Benjamin F., "Southern Gothic," *The New Encyclopedia of Southern Culture, vol. 9: Literature*, edited by M. Thomas Inge, 145-151.Chapel Hill, NC: The University of North Carolina Press, 2008.

Garner, Dwight. "Crisscrossing a Region of Strip Malls and Ghosts," *The New York Times*, April 23, 2013.

Gay, William. *The Long Home*. Denver, CO.: MacMurray & Beck, 1999.

Giroux, Henry A. *Zombie Politics and Culture in the Age of Casino Capitalism*. New York: Peter Lang, 2011.

Graham, Allison. "The South in Popular Culture." *A Companion to the Literature and Culture of the American South*, edited by Richard Gray and Owen Robinson, 335-351. Malden, MA: Blackwell Publishing, 2007.

Hall, Robert L. "Motorcycles, Hamburgers, and Lines You Can't Forget: An Interview with Barry Hannah." *Southern Scribe* 2, no. 11 (November 2001).
http://www.southernscribe.com/zine/authors/Hannah_Barry.htm

Hannah, Barry. *Yonder Stands Your Orphan*. New York: Atlantic Monthly Press, 2001.

McCarthy, Cormac. *No Country for Old Men*. New York: Alfred A. Knopf, 2005.

May, Robert E. "Fighting South." *The New Encyclopedia of Southern Culture, vol. 4: Myth, Manners, and Memory*, edited by Charles Reagan Wilson, 68-70.. Chapel Hill: The University of North Carolina Press, 2006.

O'Connor, Flannery. "The Fiction Writer & His Country," *Mystery and Manners: Occasional Prose*, edited by Sally and Robert Fitzgerald, 25-35. 1969; New York: Farrar, Straus & Giroux, 2000.

Reed, John Shelton, *Southern Folk, Plain & Fancy: Native White Social Types*. Athens: The University of Georgia Press, 1986.

Romine, Scott. "Orphans All: Reality Homesickness in *Yonder Stands Your Orphan*." *Perspectives on Barry Hannah*, edited by Martyn Bone, 161-182. Jackson, MS: University Press of Mississippi, 2007.

Savoy, Eric. "The Rise of the American Gothic." *The Cambridge Companion to Gothic Fiction*, edited by Jerrold E. Hogle, 167-188. Cambridge: Cambridge University Press, 2002.

Thompson, Tracy. *The New Mind of the South*. New York: Simon & Schuster, 2013.

Welsh, Jim. "Borderline Evil: The Dark Side of Byzantium in *No Country for Old Men*, Novel and Film." *No Country for Old Men: From Novel to Film*, edited by Lynnea Chapman King, Rick Wallach, and Jim Welsh, 73-85. Lanham, MA: Scarecrow Press, 2009.

Wilson, Charles Reagan. "Myth, Manners, and Memory." *The New Encyclopedia of Southern Culture, vol. 4: Myth, Manners, and Memory*, edited by Charles Reagan Wilson, 1-8. Chapel Hill: The University of North Carolina Press, 2006.

Woodward, Richard B. "Cormac McCarthy's Venomous Fiction," *The New York Times*, April 19, 1992, Section 6, p. 28.

Wyatt-Brown, Bertram. *Honor and Violence in the Old South*. New York: Oxford University Press, 1986.

Yaeger, Patricia. *Dirt and Desire: Reconstructing Southern Women's Writing 1930-1990*. Chicago: University of Chicago Press, 2000.

CHAPTER FIVE

JOAN WILLIAMS AND WILLIAM FAULKNER UNITED IN FICTION: THE IDIOT-CONNECTION

GÉRALD PRÉHER

"It is difficult to adjust to the fact that we are all alone.
Maybe that's why I wrote books, to cope with this frustration."
—Jeff in a letter to Amy
Joan Williams, *The Wintering*.[1]

Joan Williams's 1971 novel, *The Wintering*, depicts the relationship between an aspiring young woman writer and an older established author. Based upon Williams's bond with William Faulkner and stemming from an idea Faulkner submitted to her in 1950,[2] the book has often been used

[1] Joan Williams, *The Wintering* (1971; Baton Rouge: Louisiana State University Press, 1997), 100.

[2] See Faulkner's 29 September 1950 letter to Williams in Joseph Blotner, ed., *Selected Letters of William Faulkner* (New York: Random House: 1977), 307. Faulkner was, of course, expressing his feelings for Williams and disguised them under the veil of fiction probably because he did not want to seem too direct at that stage. The idea kept developing in his mind before Williams actually put pen to paper almost twenty years later. Faulkner felt that she should "[r]ewrite that first letter you sent me . . . This story will be a series of letters" (Ibid., 323). Even though Williams uses some letters in *The Wintering*, she did not write an epistolary novel; nonetheless, she did "rewrite" her first letter to Faulkner and it has been used by biographers ever since the novel appeared, thus turning their relationship into fiction.

by Faulkner biographers as a primary source on their intimate connection[3] that appears to have been of an intersubjective nature.[4] In *The Wintering*, Williams has Jeff Almoner, Faulkner's fictional double, write in a letter that

> *[you] gave me back what I had to have, a belief in what I was doing. I've needed someone to give something to, which was not money. I was tired of that. I needed someone saying Yes, to me, and to whom I could say it in return.*[5]

Like Almoner, Faulkner felt it was his duty to help Williams become a better writer. It might even be said that his letter to *Harper's* accompanying Williams's story "The Morning and the Evening," wedded them in the realm of fiction writing: "As is probably obvious the enclosed was written by a student of Faulkner."[6]

Of course, for a young writer from the South, the presence of Faulkner is intimidating since comments on any book published by a southern writer will be compared to his works; in Williams's case, it was even more perilous because Faulkner was there when she really started off.[7] In her letters to him, Williams mentioned the issue of influence and Faulkner told her that she should not worry too much:

> Never be afraid. Never give one Goddamn about what anybody says about the work, if you know you have done it as honestly and bravely and truly

---

[3] See for instance Stephen B. Oates, *William Faulkner: The Man and the Artist* (New York: Harper and Row, 1989) or André Bleikasten, *William Faulkner: Une Vie en romans* (Paris: Aden, 2007).

[4] I am using Gabriel Marcel's terminology from his *Être et Avoir* (Paris: Editions Aubier, 1935).

[5] Williams, *The Wintering*, 124. All the letters exchanged by Jeff and Amy, Williams'sfictional self, appear in the diegesis in italics.

[6] Blotner, op. cit., 337.

[7] Williams had already published a short story, "Rain Later," in *Mademoiselle* after winning a writing contest but "The Morning and the Evening" and the various letters that she exchanged with Faulkner show that she took writing as a serious activity at that point. About "Rain Later," Williams explains: "I wrote [it] without any instructions whatsoever about how to write a short story. I knew none of the things I learned later. . . I wrote instinctively and just as instinctively about the small place in Mississippi I visited" (quoted in Lisa C. Hickman, *William Faulkner and Joan Williams: The Romance of Two Writers*, Foreword by Richard Bausch [Jefferson, NC: McFarland, 2006] 20). In a letter to Faulkner, she writes "I want to work hard because of you" (Ibid. 25), which makes it clear that meeting him was a catalyst for her to write.

> as you could. Sure—some discerning person will holler Faulkner because there will be some Faulkner in it. Every writer is influenced by everything that ever touches him, from the telephone directory to God.[8]

As Louis D. Rubin has explained, those writing after Faulkner had to "get out from under him" and "[f]or that reason, part of their task has been and will be that of getting away from it, gaining perspective, learning to see their experience with their own eyes."[9] Faulkner's advice to Williams goes in the same direction and, writing about Jake, the main character in "The Morning and the Evening," he encourages her to

> feel [her character] from inside . . . To write him properly, you must have not instruction nor criticism, but imagination, which you have to have to invent him, and observation and experience. Which you will get partly from reading the best which others have done, and from watching people, accepting everything.[10]

Although it is obvious that she does "feel her characters from the inside," literary influences are palpable in Williams's fiction—for the sake of concision, this article will only focus on Faulkner's influence but Williams readers will also notice borrowings from Katherine Anne Porter, Carson McCullers or, among others, Eudora Welty. As Lisa C. Hickman points out in *William Faulkner and Joan Williams: The Romance of Two Writers*, "Joan read *The Sound and the Fury* [in 1949], and was swept away by the intensity of Faulkner's novel. It was her landscape, the kind of people she knew, and the emotions she experienced."[11] Williams was undoubtedly moved by Benjy Compson and she did recognize that there was a kinship between them—which it is tempting to define as an idiot

---

[8] Williams, "Faulkner's Advice to a Young Writer," *Faulkner and the Short Story: Faulkner and Yoknapatawpha, 1990*, eds., Evans Harrington and Ann J. Abadie (Jackson: University Press of Mississippi, 1992), 260.

[9] Louis D. Rubin, Jr., "The Difficulties of Being a Southern Writer Today: Or, Getting Out From Under William Faulkner," *The Journal of Southern History* 29, no. 4 (November 1963): 488.

[10] Blotner, 338.

[11] Hickman, 15. In a 1950 letter, Williams told Faulkner that for her *The Sound and the Fury* was the greatest book in the world (Hickman, 85), which probably accounts for Faulkner's decision to entrust her with the original manuscript of the book a few years later. For a detailed account of the manuscript's story, see Hickman, 120-122.

connection. Yet, re-reading Faulkner's *The Hamlet*, she suddenly realized that "Jake is not Benjy. He's Ike Snopes!"[12]

A recent collection in French,[13] analyzes the figure of the idiot as liminal. In their introduction, the editors start with etymology, explaining that in Greek *idios* refers to a singular citizen who was quite often pictured as "extraordinary" whereas in Latin, *idiotus*, designates an uneducated person and it is this meaning that most people have in mind when using the term "idiot." It is the combination of two etymologies that is used as a starting point in this collection of essays whose aim is to show that the idiot, as a literary figure, is intended to "reveal" the unforeseen reality of life.[14] This article concurs with the idea in an endeavor to show that Jake, Benjy and Ike make it possible to see the darkness of the southern way of life.

Although Williams asserts that she "was not consciously thinking of characters or situations in either *The Sound and the Fury* or *The Hamlet*,"[15] the aim of this article is to reflect upon literary filiations and by focusing on the relationship between Jake, Benjy and Ike to show that there is a deep thematic connection uniting them all.[16] Faulkner's response to "The Morning and the Evening" helps see how he read the story

---

[12] Williams, "Twenty Will Not Come Again," *The Atlantic Monthly* (May 1980): 65.

[13] *Idiots: Figures et personnages liminaires dans la littérature et les arts*, edited by Véronique Cnockaert, Bertrand Gervais and Marie Scarpa (Nancy: Presses Universitaires de Lorraine, 2012). Also see Frédérique Spill's introductory chapter in *L'Idiotie dans l'œuvre de William Faulkner* (Paris: Presses Sorbonne Nouvelle, 2009).

[14] Ibid., 6.

[15] Williams, "Twenty Will Not Come Again," op. cit., 65.

[16] Other Southern women writers have pictured idiots in their fiction. Porter's short story "He" revolves around the story of a simple-minded character and Williams once told an interviewer that Porter was her "strongest influence" (Patrick H. Samway, "Joan Williams: Struggling Fiction Writer," *America*, December 31, 1988, 545). See Porter, "He," *The Collected Stories* (New York: Harcourt Brace, 1965), 49-58. The reader might also be reminded of McCullers' mutes in *The Heart is a Lonely Hunter*. As for Welty, she does not resort to simple-minded characters much: a "little idiot nigger" is mentioned in "The Whole World Knows" but not developed as a fully-fledged character (*Stories, Essays & Memoirs*, eds., Richard Ford and Michael Kreyling [New York: Library of America, 1998] 471); and in "Asphodel," Miss Sabina is said to have power that "reached over the whole population—white and black, men and women, children, idiots, and animals—even strangers" (Ibid., 246). Interestingly, the idiot is listed after children but before animals, suggesting that though his faculties are limited he does not hold a subhuman position and is part of the community.

through the prism of his own fiction while Williams's treatment of the idiot in the novel of the same title confirms that she had learnt what Faulkner meant when he wrote that "loneliness should be a catalyst."[17]

"The Morning and the Evening": Faulknerizing Williams?

Williams showed a draft of "The Morning and the Evening" to Faulkner some time in 1950 and, as Lisa Hickman explains, it "struck a chord with [him]."[18] It focuses on Jake, a retarded mute who goes to see a movie and ends up being thrown out of the tent where it is shown because of his strange behavior. Faulkner felt there was nothing to be left out of the story but suggested that Williams "break up the idiot section into shorter paragraphs, even at times a single sentence to a paragraph, [for] it would help the effect; of his simple mental processes, his mental fumbling, his innocence. . . ."[19] Only in the *Atlantic Monthly* printing of the story do the four sections appear; neither in Williams's *The Morning and the Evening* (1961), where it became the opening chapter, nor in *Pariah and Other Stories* (1983), has the division been kept, even through the presence of blanks.

A look at the original version suggests that Faulkner was referring to the second section of the story (that runs from "Jake straightened up. . ." till ". . . 'Look at the pictures.'") and Williams did follow the suggestion that some sentences should stand out by being made into paragraphs. Thanks to this organization, the reader really gets a glimpse of Jake from the inside. Such isolated sentences very often refer to what Jake felt, understood or remembered. After the little girl sitting next to him has touched his face, the narrator observes: "Then he sat back, let himself feel again how the hand had felt: soft." The next paragraph, a short sentence, reads: "Softness he understood." This leads Jake to explore his memories: "The dark, the movie, the people around were lost to him now, while he was remembering softness."[20] This information is only shared between the narrator and the reader, thus making the people present in the scene doubly absent from the actual action.

---

[17] Blotner, 331.
[18] Hickman, 118.
[19] Faulkner quoted in Williams, "Faulkner's Advice to a Young Writer," 256.
[20] Williams, "The Morning and the Evening," *The Atlantic Monthly* (January 1952): 66.

If the first section introduces Jake as a "loony" through the townspeople's comments about him, the other three sections take the reader into the character's mind in order to suggest that anything he does is informed by past situations and personal explorations: "Some things he had learned, repeated things. And some things he knew instinctively, animal-like: tones, touches; whether they were kind, or not."[21] As is often the case in the first section of Faulkner's *The Sound and the Fury*, the narrator resorts to parataxis to "[strengthen] the impression that [the character] is at a stage between baby and young child."[22] Williams departs from Faulkner by using Jake as a focalizer and not as the narrator; she thus plays on Jake's position in the text and, by extension, within the community. He is part of and yet outside of it, which makes him a perfect observer of its customs—since he is not equipped with an analytical mind, his thoughts are generally factual and thus neutral. Jake is made to describe the unvarnished truth of the South through what Dorrit Cohn would call "narrated monologue,"[23] a technique particularly useful here since it "[suspends figural consciousness] on the threshold of verbalization."[24] Just like Faulkner's Benjy, Jake is inhabited by words, by scenes he can formulate in his mind but cannot let out of his mouth.[25] His mental confusion is thus transcribed in the text in order to point out the meaninglessness of social codes as regards mentally challenged individuals.

In one of his letters, Faulkner was concerned with the story's initial title which might have been simply "Jake":

> I don't like the title. You are writing about a human being, true. but I think the title should refer to a *condition*, some applicable quotation, like a child should lead them, though that is not quite right. Some word maybe, like Twilight, some tender word, or, for emphasis, some savage word or phrase. . .[26]

---

[21] Ibid., 66.

[22] Ineke Bockting, *Character and Personality in the Novels of William Faulkner: A Study in Psychostylistics* (New York: University Press of America, 1995), 44.

[23] Cohn defines "narrated monologue" as "a transformation of figural thought-language into the narrative language of third-person fiction" (Dorrit Cohn, *Transparent Minds: Narrative Modes for Presenting Consciousness in Fiction* [1978; Princeton: Princeton University Press, 1983] 100).

[24] Ibid., 103.

[25] I am borrowing François Pitavy's idea that Benjy is "*un être de mots*" (Le Bruit et la fureur *de William Faulkner* [Paris: Gallimard, "Foliothèque", 2001] 61).

[26] Faulkner quoted in Williams, "Faulkner's Advice to a Young Writer," 256.

Williams credits Faulkner with suggesting the final title—one he himself had thought of when working on *The Sound and the Fury* and later on when writing *The Hamlet*[27]—, "saying that the mute [...] did not know the difference between the morning and the evening."[28] The choice of the same title for her debut novel can be interpreted as a tribute to Faulkner; Williams makes use of the same kind of explanation when two characters wonder why Jake has been wandering around:

> "We just seen Jake coming out of your house, Ruth Edna, when we come by."
> "Jake?" Ruth Edna said. "I wonder why?"
> "'Cause you got his sewing, I reckon," Miss Loma said.
> "But he just brought it a while ago. I couldn't have done it yet."
> "Well, he don't know that. Jake don't know the morning from the evening."[29]

Although Williams asserts that Faulkner did not see the other chapters that eventually made it into *The Morning and the Evening*, the way she describes Faulkner's idea in "Twenty Will Not Come Again" confirms the fact that for her it became a driving metaphor: ". . . he suggested 'The Morning and the Evening' out of Genesis, when God created day and night; because to my mute Jake, all time is the same; it doesn't matter to him whether it's morning or evening."[30] If, when reading the short story, the meaning of the title is not that obvious, the novel offers several possibilities which, combined, make *The Morning and the Evening* a universal tale about difference and loneliness. The morning refers to what can be seen as opposed to the evening when everything is darker—it is all a question of light, surface and depth, exposure and secrecy.

---

[27] I am indebted to Jacques Pothier, who worked extensively on the drafts of *The Hamlet*, for this comment.

[28] Faulkner quoted in Williams, "Faulkner's Advice to a Young Writer," 256-257.

[29] Williams, *The Morning and the Evening* (New York: Atheneum, 1961), 83-84.

[30] Williams, "Twenty Will Not Come Again," 64. Faulkner said more or less the same thing about Benjy in an interview: "To that idiot, time was not a continuation, it was an instant, there was no yesterday and no tomorrow, it all is this moment, it all is [now] to him" (quoted in Bockting, *Character and Personality in the Novels of William Faulkner*, 56). It is also to be noted that Williams's final title is the same Faulkner had chosen for Ike's love story with the cow in what was to become *The Hamlet*. See Jacques Pothier's "Imagery and the Making of *The Hamlet*: Of Snopeses and Cows," *Faulkner in Venice*, eds. Rosella Mamoli Zorzi and Pia Masiero Marcolin (Venezia: Marsilio, 2000), 121.

The short story plays on these terms by insisting on Jake's emotional reactions to the film and on the notions of inside and outside that refer to his body and his surroundings: "he heard [the movie music] not with his ears, but inside him"[31]; "as always when something moved him, the music began to creep up inside him"[32]; "he felt words inside him the way he felt music"[33]; "he heard the singing inside him, smiling to himself"[34]; "With no thought left of what was inside the tent, Jake stood limply while the owner held him"[35]; "Alone, he began to call up words from way inside him"[36]; "When he saw the little house, with one lighted window, he went up to it and looked inside."[37] Put together, these sentences show that Jake's body becomes a liminal space, one that "[inspires] anguish and fear"[38]—a fact that is confirmed by the constant gaze of the owner-manager[39] or the behavior of the woman who "jerked the little girl away" and took her seat.[40] What is also stressed by the repetition of the adjective "inside" is that Jake has created a world of his own where he can give full vent to his feelings and knowledge: "He had known for a long time that he could sing. Whenever he was alone he would sing, but he kept it a secret."[41] Jake keeps his song and his emotions to himself; since he is unable to speak, he expresses himself differently by moaning or by reacting physically to his surroundings. Just like Faulkner in the Benjy section of *The Sound and the Fury*, Williams makes the situation confusing because the focalizer himself is confused[42]; Jake interprets everything in his own terms by taking into account his personal history. Like Benjy who initially observes a scene from a specific point—

---

[31] Williams, "The Morning and the Evening," 66.
[32] Ibid., 66.
[33] Ibid., 67.
[34] Ibid., 68.
[35] Ibid., 69.
[36] Ibid.
[37] Ibid.
[38] Ineke Bockting, "Haunted Borderland: Gothic Liminality in Texts of the American South," *Dynamics of the Threshold: Essays in Liminal Negotiations*, eds., Jesus Benito and Ana Manzanas, *Studies in Liminality and Literature* 5, (Madrid: The Gateway Press, 2006), 131.
[39] Williams, "The Morning and the Evening," 66.
[40] Ibid., 68.
[41] Ibid.
[42] In an introduction to the novel, Faulkner notes that the other sections of the novel were meant "to clarify" what Benjy described in the first part of the book (Faulkner, *The Sound and the Fury*, 1929, ed., David Minter [New York: Norton, 1994] 231).

"Through the fence"[43]—Jake rediscovers the world, his world, by looking at the movie screen. Both characters need mediation between the actual and the particular, between the abstract and the real that is hidden behind "black and white shadows"[44] similar to those Jake contemplates on the movie screen.

Noticeably, whenever he feels the urge to react to what he sees, Jake feels the menacing presence of the owner-manager around him. The first sentence in the story already hinted at the man's multiple roles:

> The owner-manager (who was also ticket-seller and -taker and would have been projectionist too if labor regulations hadn't forced him to hire a licensed one) didn't take his first customer for a loony, and tried to charge him full admission.[45]

The elements within parenthesis provide inside information and make it clear that the man is greedy and ambitious and that right from the start, as suggested by the negation, he was suspicious of Jake. In a letter to Williams, Faulkner had commented about first sentences in short stories and encouraged the young writer to revise it: "You have got to write the first sentence of a story so that whoever reads it will want to read the second one."[46] He recommended that she add in parentheses "'(and ticket-seller and -taker and everything else too, with the exception of the licensed projectionist whom labor union regulations compelled him to hire)'" because "it established right away the proprietor's character."[47] The *Atlantic Monthly* publication includes the brackets, but in the subsequent versions Williams did away with them and split the sentence into two; in both "The Morning and the Evening" (as reprinted in *Pariah and Other Stories*) and in the novel of the same title, the first paragraph reads:

> The owner-manager was also the ticket seller and ticket taker and would have been his own projectionist, too, if labor regulations had not forced him to hire a licensed one. He did not take his first customer for a loony and tried to charge him full admission.[48]

---

[43] Faulkner, *The Sound and the Fury*, 3.
[44] Williams, "The Morning and the Evening," 68.
[45] Ibid., 65.
[46] Blotner, 327.
[47] Williams, "Faulkner's Advice to a Young Writer," 257.
[48] Williams, *Pariah and Other Stories* (Boston: Little, Brown and Company, 1983) 3; Williams, *The Morning and the Evening*, 3.

Although the idea of accumulation remains thanks to the use of polysyndeton, the decision to have two sentences upsets the initial rhythm, making the direct cause to consequence effect Faulkner had introduced disappear. Faulkner's meddling with the text is still noticeable considering Williams's initial "The owner-manager did not take his first customer for a looney [sic]."[49] By defining the owner-manager, the story gains in power and the character's constant presence in the background points to him as an agent of the dark forces[50] that band together against Jake in the novel to come. The opposition between the sounds outside and their translation inside Jake's mind foreshadows another story, "The Sound of Silence," which was accepted by *Mademoiselle* but was not published until *Pariah and Other Stories* came out.

Short Stories in/and the Making of *The Morning in the Evening*

Just like "The Morning and the Evening," "The Sound of Silence,"[51] which became the third chapter in *The Morning and the Evening*, relies on Jake's sensibility. Describing Jake's discovery of his dead mother's body,[52] this chapter makes the dichotomy between inside and outside even more present. The first paragraph stands as a case in point worth quoting at length:

> She was dead. He knew it was death. She did not move for a very long time while he watched, and then he knew it was death. He had loved animals and they had been taken from him, but only after he had watched a long time and they had stayed still. And she was that still, like everywhere after a summer storm. He sat, and in the way that was his, after a time he said, "Ma. . . ."[53]

---

[49] Williams, "Twenty Will Not Come Again," 64.

[50] "[Jake] remembered the man who didn't want to take his dime, and saw him looking at him and laughing. So he grinned back. But the man's face went back into the dark" (Williams, "The Morning and the Evening," 66).

[51] The story being identical to the chapter in *The Morning and the Evening*, all the references are to the novel.

[52] The previous chapter already foreshadowed the death of Jake's mother by recounting how one day she found herself trapped in the "dark cool cellar in the earth" (Williams, *The Morning and the Evening*, 22).

[53] Ibid., 44.

The focus of the sentences alternates between the mother and the son, suggesting a back and forth movement: Jake watches his mother and then comes to a conclusion. This idea is reinforced by the numerous repetitions that flesh out the fact presented in the paratactic first two sentences. The situation calls to mind George Didi-Huberman's theory that "what we look at only has value—is only alive—in our eyes because it stares at us in the face" which he derives from James Joyce's "ineluctable modality of the visible" in *Ulysses*.[54] For Jake what is "visible" is that his mother is "still" which brings yet another image, that of dead animals; his love for his mother only filters through the adjective he associates with them. Jake's behavior echoes Michel Foucault's comment in *Madness and Civilization* that "the disturbance of his reason restored the madman to the immediate kindness of nature by a return to animality."[55] His simple frame of mind is thus exposed at the same time as it exposes him to loss and loneliness.

Likewise in the opening chapter of the book, when he sees a man stroking a girl's hair on the screen, memories of his late beloved cow surface: "He watched the stroking . . . —soft, soft, he knew remembering Sarah Jane. He began to ache remembering Sarah Jane."[56] Faulkner's conception of literary influence is verified here since Jake, just like Ike Snopes in *The Hamlet*, feels for a cow, speaks to it.[57] In both cases, the mute and the cow seem apt to "understand" each other as they somehow share a common language: moaning. In addition, Sarah Jane "was the only one who would listen" while everyone else tried to hush him. Afraid that something more than just stroking the animal might be happening between Jake and the cow, his mother "would take him away"[58] and never would he be able to express the depth of his feelings for the only being who really understood him. The townsmen reacted much the same way when, seeing how faithful their dogs were to them, Jake would "tell them how he wanted a dog, too."[59] Aloneness is imposed upon Jake who is forever

[54] Georges Didi-Huberman, *Ce que nous voyons, ce qui nous regarde* (1991; Paris: Les Editions de Minuit, 2001), 9, my translation.

[55] Michel Foucault, *Madness and Civilization: A History of Insanity in the Age of Reason* (1961; translated by Richard Howard; New York: Random House, 1979), 75.

[56] Williams, *The Morning and the Evening*, 16.

[57] Faulkner, *Snopes: The Hamlet, The Town, The Mansion*, 1940, 1957, 1959, Introduction by George Garrett (New York: Modern Library, 1994), 160. Unlike Faulkner, though, Williams does not go as far as using an animal as focalizer.

[58] Williams, *The Morning and the Evening*, 16.

[59] Ibid., 12.

misunderstood; he watches other people's happiness without being able to share in it.

All Jake seems to "know" is loss and, like Faulkner, it seems that Williams is "interested in the relationship of the idiot to the world that he [is] in but would never be able to cope with and just where could he get the tenderness, the help, to shield his innocence."[60] The animal world offers itself as a friendlier place for such characters. In *The Hamlet*, it is only after a long description of Ike and his "female" other, that the identity of the couple is eventually revealed: the reader first finds out that the unnamed he in the text "[sees] nothing but the cow"[61] before Ike attempts to pronounce his name without much success.[62] The order in which the characters' identity appears is of prime importance since it suggests both an origin and a destination: the cow makes it possible for Ike to name himself partly because he has found his true self in that unusual love.[63]

Unfortunately for Williams's Jake, intimate unity is never achieved and Jake is unable to name himself: the sounds that come out of his mouth, though they are meaningful to him and to the reader who has access to his thoughts, never signify anything for the members of the community. Because they do not understand, some men mock Jake saying "'You ain't crazy, are you, Jake?'" and, since he cannot reply, others do it for him: "'Naw, but you ain't far from it are you, Jake?'"[64] Joan Williams has explained that her story "was sparked by a retarded man in my grandmother's town. People teased him by saying 'You're not crazy, are you?' And he'd reply, 'Naw. But me ain't far from it.' How, I wanted to know, did people not know his feelings were hurt?"[65] Contrary to Jake who cannot respond and does not seem to take any notice of what is being said about him, the man in Williams's recollection can speak and he plays along. By presenting the world through innocent eyes, Williams reveals the violence of human nature and paradoxically speaks through her mute character. Talking about *The Sound and the Fury*, she once confessed: "what had moved me in [Benjy's section] was his inarticulateness, because

---

[60] Faulkner quoted in Bockting, *Character and Personality in the Novels of William Faulkner*, 49.
[61] Faulkner, *Snopes: The Hamlet, The Town, The Mansion*, 160.
[62] Ibid., 161.
[63] For a detailed analysis of this scene, see Frédérique Spill, *L'Idiotie dans l'œuvre de William Faulkner* (Paris: Presses Sorbonne Nouvelle, 2009), 161-164.
[64] Williams, *The Morning and the Evening*, 49.
[65] Williams, "Twenty Will Not Come Again," 64.

I felt it to be my own"[66]—with *The Morning and the Evening*, she uses a protagonist who occupies the center from the margin.[67]

After his mother's death, Jake fails to formulate his inner pain in words; he seeks comfort by joining the chickens in the yard, picks up one, "[holds] its soft yellow roundness close to him [...]. And he [tries] to tell the animal in great dry sobs, but he knew no words for loss."[68] Frédérique Spill has shown that "if he is unable to speak, the idiot is nonetheless equipped with a voice."[69] Focusing on quotations drawn from *The Sound and the Fury*, she aptly demonstrates that Benjy's moaning could be understood as an illustration of the title and of the impossibility of formulating the inacceptable. Indeed, "moaning" and "mourning" seem to go hand in hand as the odd conversation between Caddy and Frony in the Benjy section of the novel suggests[70]; paronomasia is brought into play to emphasize the characters' difficulty communicating but it is also implied that for Benjy "moaning" and "mourning" sound the same and are therefore equivalent—a conclusion that Joan Williams might have reached as well when she designed Jake.

The oxymoronic title of Williams's story, "The Sound of Silence," seems to introduce a totally different perspective from Faulkner's. After Jake's discovery, silence imposes itself: "[his mother] did not answer. She had not answered all morning. When he opened his eyes to daytime, for the first time in the forty years of his life he had not heard her in the house."[71] The use of negations together with the idea of a new day beginning announces the future that lies ahead and the human loneliness Jake will experience from that point onwards. When the man who brings the ice appears—another symbol of the coldness that has set in and will continue to develop as the body of Jake's mother is taken away—, all the references to silence and sounds create an oppressive atmosphere: "In the silence afterward, Jake could hear the man's heavy breathing"; "Jake could hear the alarm clock ticking in there. Then he could hear the heavy steps of the man."[72] The narrator places the emphasis on actions that are

---

[66] Ibid., 65.

[67] François Pitavy sees the idiot as the "organization principle" in *The Hamlet* but he notes that in *The Sound and the Fury* everything revolves around Caddy, not around Benjy ("Idiotie et idéalisme: Réflexion sur l'idiot faulknérien," *Études anglaises* 35.4 [October-December 1982]: 414).

[68] Williams, *The Morning and the Evening*, 45.

[69] Spill, 55, my translation.

[70] Faulkner, *The Sound and the Fury*, 24.

[71] Williams, *The Morning and the Evening*, 44.

[72] Ibid., 55.

connected to life ("breathing") and time (reference to the clock) but also on the heaviness of the situation, which filters through the portrayal of the intruder. The paratactic style gives the text a specific rhythm that mirrors the progression of the man towards the house; it is as if a film were playing in Jake's mind, diverting his attention from what is really at stake. He starts picturing the scene that leads to the man's discovery of his mother's lifeless body, focusing on the emptiness that can be felt in the landscape:

> Then the man was on the front porch. He heard the door slam behind him. And he knew how it would look: the empty porch, the stilled swing, ahead the empty road and quiet flat land; and the field, still too, rising in the distance to a road where you could see the white steeple of the church. He thought he heard a bird sing, and he could feel the warmth of the day flush on his face as he knew the man could; sweat stood out on his forehead. Presently he heard the man open the door to re-enter the house, and he stood up and went down the hall, meaning neither to be quiet nor to make noise, but the man did not hear him. He was in her room, bending over the bed. Jake stood outside the door, watching. He heard the man's heavy intake of breath, watched as he held her arm a moment, then let it fall quickly. He drew the sheet up over her face.[73]

The house soon fills with people who are concerned with Jake's situation. After his mother's body is taken away, the women see to it that Jake gets something to eat but as evening is drawing near, everyone is heading home, leaving Jake alone. Once again, it is the quietness of the outside that attracts Jake's attention[74] while inside the clock is still ticking, making the passage of time more difficult to bear: "in the silence of the house he heard only the clock in the bedroom and the sound of his own breathing. He was alone and he knew that."[75] The "sound of silence" is what defines Jake's life in the early days following his mother's passing; it constitutes what Julia Kristeva would call "the imaginary or symbolic level"[76] and makes it possible for Jake to recover his mother and deny his

[73] Ibid., 55-56.
[74] Ibid., 64.
[75] Ibid., 65. Williams uses the same kind of imagery in "No Love for the Lonely," a short story which focuses on other characters present in the novel. It describes the effects of Ruth Edna's death on her brother who, just like Jake, finds himself alone and helpless: "[h]e tried to hear in the silence that welcomed him an echo, a voice from the past, tried to make his memories bring the house alive, but he could not" (Williams, *Pariah and Other Stories*, 73).
[76] Julia Kristeva, *Black Sun: Depression and Melancholia* (1987; translated by Leon Roudiez; New York: Columbia, 1992), 40.

loss. The narrator insists on the fact that the "sounds" that can be heard do not constitute any act of speech, instead, they refer to Jake's "*own* breathing" or to his "*own* noise"—as though he were trying to fill up the emptiness that his mother's death had left by affirming his presence. His reaction illustrates Kristeva's theory of the "impossible *mourning for the maternal object*"[77] for Jake never severed his bond with his mother and he never entered language. The symbolic refuge Jake builds for himself soon wears out and his sounds no longer fill the surrounding silence. One night, the nature of his estrangement comes to the surface:

> He lay awake as the night and its silence deepened. He had always known silence, but suddenly he was afraid of it. He sat up, startled, and with one terrified, but reassuring cry, called out at the top of his lungs, telling them all, telling everybody, the one thing in the world he did know fully: that as deep as his own silence was, it was nowhere near so deep as hers.[78]

Listening to the sounds from the outside, to fill the emptiness and the silence inside him, has proved unsuccessful. The different stages Jake goes through in this chapter illustrate what Freud has suggested in "Mourning and Melancholia": the completion of the mourning process is not possible if the subject does not go through a period of melancholia.[79] The fact that silence is associated with both the night and the mother seems to indicate the darkness that is now coloring Jake's thoughts; the absence of a referent for the pronouns "hers" confirms that his mourning is now over, an element that is confirmed in the rest of the novel from which the mother—or memories of her—are totally absent.

Critics who exclusively focused on Williams's relationship with Faulkner caused her work to be forgotten. Faulkner scholars recognize her name but not many have looked into her fiction. A close study of Williams's early works reveals that long before the publication of the semi-autobiographical novel, *The Wintering*, the special bond she shared with William Faulkner could be felt in her choice of a retarded character whose predicament resembles those of Benjy Compson and Ike Snopes very closely. *The Morning and the Evening* might be read as a tribute to a mentor who, in their early exchanges, reminded Williams that "the point

---

[77] Ibid., 9.

[78] Williams, *The Morning and the Evening*, 76.

[79] See Sigmund Freud, "Mourning and Melancholia", translated by Joan Riviere, *General Psychological Theory*, ed., Philip Rieff (New York: Collier, 1963), 164-179.

of writing […] was to make something passionate and moving and true."[80] One should hope that readers will soon discover what Faulkner meant when he classified Williams's first published story ("Rain Later") in that category. Although Williams dedicated her sole short story collection to Faulkner, the rare interviews that focus on her works and not on her personal life do not include any reference to her mentor: she obviously wanted to do away with him—maybe because her writing is ample proof of Faulkner's lasting presence? The idiot-connection is the best evidence.

Works Cited

Bleikasten, André. *William Faulkner: Une Vie en romans*. Paris: Aden, 2007.

Blotner, Joseph, ed. *Selected Letters of William Faulkner*. New York: Random House: 1977.

Bockting, Ineke. *Character and Personality in the Novels of William Faulkner: A Study in Psychostylistics*. New York: University Press of America, 1995.

—. "Haunted Borderland: Gothic Liminality in Texts of the American South." *Dynamics of the Threshold: Essays in Liminal Negotiations*, edited by Jesus Benito and Ana Manzanas, 39-54. *Studies in Liminality and Literature* 5. Madrid: The Gateway Press, 2006.

Cnockaert, Véronique, Bertrand Gervais and Marie Scarpa, eds. *Idiots: Figures et personnages liminaires dans la littérature et les arts*. Nancy: Presses Universitaires de Lorraine, 2012.

Cohn, Dorrit. *Transparent Minds: Narrative Modes for Presenting Consciousness in Fiction*. 1978. Princeton: Princeton University Press, 1983.

Didi-Huberman, Georges. *Ce que nous voyons, ce qui nous regarde*. 1991. Paris: Les Editions de Minuit, 2001.

Faulkner, William. *The Sound and the Fury*, edited by David Minter. 1929; New York: Norton, 1994.

—. *Snopes: The Hamlet, The Town, The Mansion*. 1940, 1957, 1959. Introduction by George Garrett. New York: Modern Library, 1994.

Foucault, Michel. *Madness and Civilization: A History of Insanity in the Age of Reason*. 1961. Translated by Richard Howard. New York: Random House, 1979.

[80] Williams, "Twenty Will Not Come Again," 64; Blotner, 297.

Freud, Sigmund. "Mourning and Melancholia." Translated by Joan Riviere. *General Psychological Theory*, edited by Philip Rieff, 164-179. New York: Collier, 1963.

Hickman, Lisa C. *William Faulkner and Joan Williams: The Romance of Two Writers*. Foreword by Richard Bausch. Jefferson, NC: McFarland, 2006.

Kristeva, Julia. *Black Sun: Depression and Melancholia*. 1987. Translated by Leon Roudiez. New York: Columbia, 1992.

Marcel, Gabriel. *Être et Avoir*. Paris: Editions Aubier, 1935.

Oates, Stephen B. *William Faulkner: The Man and the Artist*. New York: Harper and Row, 1989.

Pitavy, François. "Idiotie et idéalisme: Réflexion sur l'idiot faulknérien." *Études anglaises* 35, no. 4 (October-December 1982): 408-419.

—. Le Bruit et la fureur *de William Faulkner*. Paris: Gallimard, "Foliothèque", 2001.

Pothier, Jacques. "Imagery and the Making of *The Hamlet*: Of Snopeses and Cows." *Faulkner in Venice*, edited by Rosella Mamoli Zorzi and Pia Masiero Marcolin, 113-127. Venezia: Marsilio, 2000.

Porter, Katherine Anne. *The Collected Stories*. New York: Harcourt Brace, 1965.

Rubin, Louis D., Jr. "The Difficulties of Being a Southern Writer Today: Or, Getting Out From Under William Faulkner." *The Journal of Southern History* 29, no. 4 (November 1963): 486-494.

Samway, Patrick H. "Joan Williams: Struggling Fiction Writer." *America*, December 31, 1988, 544-545, 549.

Spill, Frédérique. *L'Idiotie dans l'œuvre de William Faulkner*. Paris: Presses Sorbonne Nouvelle, 2009.

Welty, Eudora. *Stories, Essays & Memoirs*, edited by Richard Ford and Michael Kreyling. New York: Library of America, 1998.

Williams, Joan. "The Morning and the Evening." *The Atlantic Monthly* (January 1952): 65-69.

—. *The Morning and the Evening*. New York: Atheneum, 1961.

—. "Twenty Will Not Come Again." *The Atlantic Monthly* (May 1980): 58-65.

—. *The Wintering*. 1971. Baton Rouge: Louisiana State University Press, 1997.

—. *Pariah and Other Stories*. Boston: Little, Brown and Company, 1983.

—. "Faulkner's Advice to a Young Writer." *Faulkner and the Short Story: Faulkner and Yoknapatawpha, 1990*, edited by Evans Harrington and Ann J. Abadie, 253-262. Jackson: University Press of Mississippi, 1992.

CHAPTER SIX

SUSAN P. GRIGSBY AND THE PSYCHOLOGICAL DIMENSION OF DISEASE AND DEATH IN ANTEBELLUM AND CIVIL WAR KENTUCKY

SUSANNA DELFINO

Whoever has visited Monticello, Thomas Jefferson's residence in Virginia, must not have failed to be struck by the shortness of the beds: too short even for eighteenth century Americans, whose stature is known to have been much lower than that of their descendants of the following century. And it has probably been with surprise that the visitors have learnt that their ancestors did not need longer beds because of the extreme diffusion of respiratory conditions which forced them to sleep with their backs upright and propped up by many pillows. The mansion's parlor has most certainly offered another occasion of astonishment at the realization that the music stand or reading desk looking-like pieces of furniture placed all around the fireplace were not at all connected with entertainment, being in fact adjustable screens people used to prevent the thick layer of makeup, that most of them put on their faces to cover the indelible marks of small pox, from melting with the heat. These simple examples aptly illustrate how even those who occupied the higher rungs of southern society could not escape the physical debilitations and disfigurements produced by diseases of various descriptions.

Disease and death were part and parcel of the lives of eighteenth and nineteenth century Americans, to the point of being considered normal occurrences. As shown by the mortality statistics of the federal census, even in the last two decades of the antebellum era the death rate was still very high in the United States, and women and children overwhelmingly contributed to the appalling figure. While the vast majority of casualties among females aged between twenty and forty was related to childbearing and its consequences, their offspring did not stand better chances of survival. Seventeen to twenty percent of all infants reported by the 1850 census died under the age of one and, much disquietingly, the death rate among children under five rose from thirty-eight to forty-three percent during the following decade.[1]

Because southern women bore more children than their northern counterparts—about eight on the average, with peaks of up to fourteen—they were particularly exposed to life danger connected with childbearing and its aftermath. But even when a woman had a smooth pregnancy, delivery could give rise to complications that caused fevers, chills, headaches, and pains of different sorts for several months thereafter. Reportedly, closely repeated pregnancies almost unavoidably resulted in a woman's progressive physical decay and, with time, might engender forms of permanent invalidity.[2]

Childbearing and nursing constituted a major challenge for southern white women of every social class but must have been absolutely dramatic for working class females, who could neither afford extended periods of rest nor possessed the financial means to secure domestic help.

Although elite women in general could find relief and support in the services of nurses and servants—mostly slaves—the lot of the mistress of a plantation or large farming estate was much more critical than that of her urban peer. The biographies of thousands of such women illustrate that, far from being the worriless and pampered creatures portrayed by the legend of the Old South, they bore instead heavy responsibilities not only in the running of their households, but also in the management of their estates.[3] No matter how many domestic servants they could avail themselves of, illness, whether or not connected with pregnancy, was extremely distressful for them, especially when their households comprised several small children. Anxieties multiplied when husbands were away attending to their businesses or political commitments. Because plantation

---

[1] Richard W. Wertz and Dorothy Wertz, *Living-In: A History of Childbirth in America* (New York: Free Press, 1977), 108; Judith W. Leavitt, *Brought to Bed: Childbearing in America, 1750-1950* (New York: Oxford University Press, 1986), 79.

[2] Leigh Fought, *Southern Womanhood and Slavery: A Biography of Louisa S. McCord, 1810-1879* (Columbia, MO: University of Missouri Press, 2003), 5.

[3] Anne Firor Scott, *The Southern Lady: From Pedestal to Politics, 1830-1930* (Chicago: University of Chicago Press, 1970), 23-44; Catherine Clinton, *Plantation Mistress: Woman's World in the Old South* (New York: Pantheon, 1982), 10-35; Catherine Clinton, *Tara Revisited: Women, War, & the Plantation Legend* (New York: Abbeville Press, 1995), 27-49; Elizabeth Fox-Genovese, *Within the Plantation Household: Black and White Women of the Old South* (Chapel Hill, NC: University of North Carolina Press, 1988), 48-51.

mistresses were expected to act as *alter egos* during their husbands' usually frequent and sometimes long absences from home, un-wellness and physical weakness often made them feel inadequate to cope with redoubled duties and responsibilities, and easily generated in them frustration and a sense of helplessness.[4]

Aware of the heavy toll in children's lives that apparently curable but often insidious affections exacted, such women also harbored constant anxieties about the well-being of their offspring, and the eventual loss of one child or more of them began to undermine their psychical balance, leading to the insurgence of severe nervous conditions that might have precise physical consequences. The above circumstances combined to make the existence of a plantation mistress a miserable one. Such was the case with Susan P. Grigsby who lost five of the seven children she bore between 1851 and 1861 before any of them reached the age of ten. Lilie Shelby, born in early December 1860, survived only twenty-five days. Four more died from diphtheria in October 1862.[5]

Due to its unhealthier climate compared with the northern United States, the incidence of disease and death was particularly heavy in the South. Yet, while epidemics such as cholera, typhus, or yellow fever have somewhat intrigued historians, the vast array of ordinary but no less potentially lethal ailing conditions that constantly troubled and even threatened the lives of southerners, has not elicited special attention. Affections such as croup, pneumonia, bronchitis, enteritis, or diphtheria could in fact be as mortal as epidemics, and took a heavy toll in human lives among white and colored alike. Ample testimony of their ravages was left by middle and upper class whites, and overwhelmingly by females who, because of the risks connected with their reproductive function and their attachment to their offspring, were particularly sensitive to the always impending menace of death. Also, women were more likely than men to keep a diary, a journal, or entertain correspondence with relatives and friends to fill their hours of solitude, especially at the end of the day, if they had dispatched their duties.

The South could not certainly boast a healthy climate, especially in summertime, which was in fact commonly referred to as "the sickly season."[6] From June through September, extreme heat and humidity favored the proliferation of all sorts of bugs and bacteria that infested its vast, un-reclaimed swampy areas and were the carriers of infective

---

[4] Fox-Genovese, *Within the Plantation Household*, 205-6.

[5] Susan P. Grigsby Correspondence, 1861-62. Grigsby Family Papers. Filson Historical Society, Louisville, Kentucky. Hereafter, FHS.

[6] John Irwin, Letters 1832. FHS.

diseases such as malaria and typhus that people contracted either through sting, water drinking, or food. Some of them, like cholera, small pox, and yellow fever were highly contagious, and quickly developed into true and proper epidemics. Their frequency and aggressiveness were especially severe in the Lower South, prompting many to avoid potential contamination by temporarily migrating somewhere farther north. And they were not only upper or middle class people who could take the opportunity to either visit with family living at less inclement latitudes—whether the Upper South, the old Northwest, or the Mid-Atlantic States—or to spend an extended vacation time at one of the several spas dotting the Atlantic states from Virginia to New York state. Thousands of artisans and common laborers also flocked to the Upper South in search of a seasonal job and, thanks to its easy accessibility through the Mississippi river and the rather dynamic market for free labor, Kentucky was a most favorite destination of theirs. The city of Louisville, which was located right at the falls of the Ohio, received thousands and thousands of such seasonal migrants. In 1853, no less an authority than statistician and superintendent of the federal census James D. B. De Bow estimated that at least fifty thousand people visited Louisville each year from downriver. Because of its burgeoning commercial and industrial economy, the Falls City offered a good number of them a variety of employment opportunities. A few years later, John F. Jefferson, the son of a wealthy merchant in dry goods and provisions noted in his diary: "large masses are constantly passing the city … all in high spirits in expectation of immediate employment." Those who were unable to seize one in the city, most likely unskilled people with an agricultural background, fanned out across the state in search of a job on a farm, plantation, or cattle raising estate. However not devoid of difficulties and uncertainties, summer life in Kentucky must have felt like heaven to those seasonal migrants compared with the unbearably humid heat of Louisiana or Mississippi.[7]

Although relatively less recurrent and destructive than those that mangled the Lower South, infectious diseases did not spare Kentucky either, especially during the summer, when the rivers' water level lowered so much as to create swampy areas where mosquitoes and other dangerous insects could thrive and feast.[8] Threats to people's health were not however confined to the "sickly season." Among the many testimonies available, the correspondence of Susan P. Grigsby is particularly revealing not only of the incidence of disease and death in one of the most

[7] John Jefferson Diary, February 6, 1857. FHS.; Mina Conrad Hegewald, "Louisville Notes," 1880. FHS.

[8] Horace Carter, Letters, August 2, 1838. FHS.

economically developed among the slave states, but also of their physical and psychical impact on a southern upper class woman.

* * *

The grand-daughter of Isaac Shelby, one of the founders of Kentucky and its first governor, Susan had been born in February 1830 at Traveller's Rest, Lincoln county, being the second child of Alfred, one of Isaac's sons, and of Virginia Hart. Having inherited the Shelbys' mansion, which they considered the shrine of the family prestige, the young couple cherished hopes to improve Traveller's Rest through hard work and a wise management of the estate. Unfortunately, their dreams shipwrecked only four years after their marriage, when Alfred accidentally died during a hunting party leaving his twenty-three-year-old spouse with three small children to raise, and pregnant with a fourth one.[9]

By the time of Alfred's death Susan was only two, but the tragic loss of her young father deeply affected her psychological development. The untimely death of her infant sister Sarah, which occurred only a few months after her birth, in 1833, further aggravated Susan, pervading her with a sense of the fragility and precariousness of human existence. She therefore developed a desperate need to be constantly reassured that, although deprived of its male head, hers was still a "real" family on which she could count for loving attention, protection, and support. In the simple but absolutely consistent reasoning of a child, Susan understood *family* as the outcome of the special bonds of affection tying people of the same blood who live under the same roof, that are cemented over time by the sharing of memories in shared places that make them feel individual parts of an indivisible whole. Home was therefore as important to her as familial attachments.[10]

Much to Susan's dismay her young, widowed mother was however determined not to surrender the administration of her estate in the hands of its testamentary executors. Virginia Hart Shelby thus courageously decided to turn herself into a businesswoman to safeguard her and her offspring's inheritance from potential encroachments, and with a view to possibly increasing the family assets. Such a challenge entailed frequent travel, precisely as any male in her position would have been forced to take. As a

[9] Dorman Fredrickson, *The Prestons of Smithfield and Greenfield in Virginia* (Louisville, KY: Filson Club Publications, 2nd ser., n. 3, 1982), 256; Archibald Henderson, "Isaac Shelby: Revolutionary Patriot and Border Hero," *The North Carolina Booklet* 16 (1917), 109-14.

[10] Susan P. Grigsby Correspondence, 1843-45. Grigsby Family Papers. FHS.

child, Susan Shelby deeply resented her mother's absences, and even more so when, as an adolescent, she was enrolled in a Lexington female school while her two brothers, Isaac and Alfred, were forwarded to an educational plan appropriate for boys. Susan would not resign herself to this new reality and, from Lexington, would write her mother letters in which she insistently asked when she would go see her. Virginia's visits to her daughter were in fact rare and Susan often inquired about her with Mr. Burns, the school principal, whose invariable answer was that her mother's inability to come see her was due to her extensive business commitments—which was probably true. Yet, the young girl could not stop herself from conveying to her mother her nostalgia for home and yearning for the next family reunion. By mid-September 1842, only a month or so past the summer break, she wrote her: "I suppose you had too much business on hand just now … I certainly look for you in a month or two," most probably looking forward to the Christmas holidays, when the family would gather again at Traveller's Rest.[11]

It was probably in reaction to her unconscious fear of not having her mother's unconditional attention that, during adolescence, Susan developed an almost morbid attachment to her, that she manifested in a compulsion to let her know, time and again, how much she loved her, and how completely she relied on her for guidance and advice. Such an attitude accompanied Susan into adulthood, and did not subside even after she had formed a family of her own. Virginia Shelby, on her part, was much concerned about her daughter's extreme psychological dependency on her, and became convinced that exposure to social and cultural environments more stimulating than Danville's would have helped Susan gain more self-reliance and autonomy. So, once Susan had graduated from the Danville Female Academy, in 1845, Virginia agreed that she joined her first cousin Sarah Gibson in attending a very exclusive French school in Philadelphia. Although reluctantly, Susan had to abide to her mother's decision. Despite the new experience in a large, eastern city pleased her a lot, Susan continued to write yearning letters to her mother and brothers. Finally, in late 1846, she got word from her brother Isaac that their mother contemplated remarrying. The news deeply unsettled Susan Shelby, and prompted her to immediately return to Kentucky.[12]

Her preoccupations were manifold. Firstly, her mother's marriage would have implied the loss of identity of her nuclear family, which would have merged with that of the betrothed, Robert J. Breckinridge, the more

---

[11] Susan P. Shelby Correspondence, 1842. Grigsby Family Papers. FHS.
[12] Susan P. Grigsby Correspondence, 1845-46. Grigsby Family Papers. FHS.

so on account that she herself and both of her brothers were still minors. In this connection, she wondered what would have become of Traveller's Rest during her brother Isaac's minority. Secondly, because Robert was a widower with several children, some of whom still in infancy, Susan feared that Virginia's energies and thoughts would have been almost completely absorbed by their care, to her own and her brothers' disadvantage. More so should her mother have borne Robert children of their own. Lastly, intimations that Breckinridge's brilliant public record as a Presbyterian minister, intellectual, and outspoken social reformer did not seem to be matched by impeccable private behavior because of his well-known intractable and often choleric temper, much disquieted Susan. The two were however deeply taken with each other and, in spite of all attempts made by Virginia's kin to dissuade her, they were finally married in April 1847.[13]

Susan might have chosen to continue her studies in Philadelphia, but was afraid that prolonged separation from her mother might lessen the intensity of her attachment to her daughter at a time when she was about to start a new family. The only possibility she foresaw to avoid such an unfortunate occurrence was to stand by her side and become Virginia's reference figure for material help and moral support. Consequently, after the wedding was celebrated, she moved into the Breckinridges' household, where she soon felt uncomfortable, most probably due to her perceived loss of identification with her nuclear family of such prestige as the Shelbys. Because of her minority age, Susan was however unable to change her situation. So, she looked for respite in travel. When her mother prematurely gave birth to Virginia, her first child by Breckinridge, Susan had just come back from Memphis, where she had been visiting with some friends.[14]

Despite her serious intention to help her mother with the caring of her troop of step-children, and with the nursing of little Virginia, Susan Shelby was not happy and continued to feel somewhat out of place in her new home. Mindful of the life experience of her mother who, having been widowed at age twenty-three, had to take on the responsibility of

---

[13] Isaac Shelby, Jr. to Susan P. Shelby, March 7, 1846. Susan P. Grigsby Correspondence, 1846-47; Letitia Wallace to Susan P. Shelby. March 6, 1846 or 1847. Grigsby Family Papers. FHS. Robert J. Breckinridge Papers, 1846-47. Library of Congress, Manuscript Division, Washington, D. C.; James C. Klotter, *The Breckinridges of Kentucky, 1760-1981* (Lexington, KY: The University Press of Kentucky, 1981), 53-58.

[14] Robert J. Breckinridge to Tobias Gibson, February 11, 1848. John W. Jones Papers. University of Kentucky Lexington, Special Collections.

managing the estate for her own and her children's sake alike, immolating her youth on the altar of family, Susan perceived marriage as a source of pain, sorrow, and never ending worries, rather than of joy and self-gratification. Her negative attitude was reinforced by the observation of Virginia's progressive physical and mental decay. Consequently, she joined many other young ladies of the Old South in indefinitely postponing the conclusion of a matrimonial alliance, and graciously waived the courtship of her suitors.[15]

Following the untimely death of her two brothers, which occurred in the span of a single month in December 1848, Susan slowly began to develop an albeit unconscious desire to form a family of her own. During a visit with her Gibson relatives in Louisiana, she met a handsome and fascinating Virginian by the name of John Warren Grigsby, and fell madly in love with him, fully reciprocated. Suspicions that he might be a dower hunter were reinforced by the fact that nothing was known about his family background, and he seemed to be of modest means. In spite of all obstacles, Susan and John were however married on November 5, 1850.[16]

A few months later, the Grigsbys left for an extended honeymoon in Europe, where John had spent some time earlier in the diplomatic service of the United States. They travelled extensively across France, England, and Italy and their first son, Alfred, was born in Florence in October 1851. Susan thought that all that was splendid, but was also conscious that the rosy period she was enjoying was not bound to last forever, and that the reality of married life was much different from the dream-like experience she was having in Europe. Cousin Susan Wallace, to whom she had conveyed such feelings in a letter written when she had but recently become aware of being pregnant, so tried to reassure her: "Your honey moon I trust will not be the end of the pleasure you speak of but my sincere wish is that however much happiness you have heretofore enjoyed it may be increased then fold in time to come."[17] However, if on the one hand Susan dreaded the responsibilities awaiting her upon return to the States, on the other, she longed to see her mother again, and was eager to

---

[15] W.C. Anderson to Susan P. Shelby, July 26, 1849. Grigsby Family Papers. FHS; Fought, *Southern Womanhood and Slavery*, 5.

[16] Fayette County, Marriage Records, 1850. Kentucky Department of Libraries and Archives, Frankfort, Kentucky.

[17] Susan Wallace to Susan P. Grigsby, March 9, 1851. Grigsby Family Papers. FHS.

resettle at Traveller's Rest, of which she had become the only heiress in consequence of her two brothers' death.[18]

In June 1852 the Grigsbys were finally back in Kentucky, and Susan was thrilled at the idea of restoring the Shelbys' ancestral home to its past splendor, and making it again a lively center of refined social and cultural life. Disappointments were not late to arrive and, in spite of her ambitions and expectations, Susan found herself living in near-isolation, largely ostracized by her peers in the neighborhood, most of whom perceived John Grigsby as an outsider of obscure origins who lacked the credentials to be admitted in the circles of polite society. Even some old friends and relatives who happened to be in the area avoided paying a visit or dropping a note. Susan was dismayed and deeply hurt by such behaviors that suggested to her the unpleasant reality that, in the absence of surviving male descendants, the name of the Shelbys did not command anymore the consideration and prestige it had long enjoyed. Although disappointingly, Susan was learning a lesson: despite her being a Shelby, her gender and the fact that she had married a stranger with no pedigree made the legacy of Traveller's Rest and its old sway largely irrelevant to many of her same social standing. Rather haughtily, Susan hastily classified them all as people unworthy of her attention, but in her heart she was much disquieted at the realization that the past could not be resurrected. Yet, instinctively, she continued to pursue her private dream, plunging herself headlong in the renovation and refurbishing of the old mansion.[19]

Susan P. Grigsby rightly perceived isolation as major hindrance to the attainment of a modicum of happiness. Although Danville was only a four or five hours' ride away, and Lexington a full day from Traveller's Rest, opportunities to see her mother were becoming increasingly rare. In 1852, Virginia had in fact three little ones to nurse, and Susan was pregnant for a second time. Such circumstances resulted in a major curtailment of either woman's freedom of movement. To make up for their insatiable desire to talk and share, they therefore relied on trustworthy slaves to exchange almost daily messages, but also to supply Susan with the variety of goods

[18] Fredrickson, The Prestons, 256-57; State of Kentucky, Court of Appeals, Alfred Shelby's Will. R. J. Breckinridge Papers. Library of Congress, Manuscript Division, Washington, D.C.

[19] Susan P. Grigsby Correspondence, 1852-53 and undated letters. Grigsby Family Papers. FHS.

and articles she needed, or wanted, from foods to tableware, and to fabrics.[20]

Christmas Day of 1853 epitomized the extent of the loneliness Susan would have experienced in the years to come. On that "wretched day so cold & windy," Mr. Grigsby was forced to leave home on some urgent business. On account of her husband's chronic respiratory problems, perhaps bronchial asthma, she was much worried about his health. With two infants to tend, she could not even go to church on such an important religious holiday. Yet, in the hope that better times would come for her family, she declared herself contented with "reading, writing and the babies [who] are all inexhaustible sources of enjoyment…"[21]

During the following six years, Susan's expectations to rationally organize the management of her household by wisely combining the work of domestic slaves with that of a white housekeeper seemed at times to be in reach of fulfilment. Yet, a variety of adverse circumstances repeatedly undercut her endeavors. Discouraged at seeing the state of disarray in which her house was lying, and despairing of any possibility to handle the situation, she sadly commented to her mother: "I have determined to let the house and kitchen take care of themselves..," and, "I wish I had a quiet respectable woman staying with me who would attend the children & the house—for I have never been in such a predicament before."[22]

Between mid-1853 and mid-1854, Susan Grigsby enjoyed a period of relative respite from the discomforts of childbearing. Yet, she regularly suffered from many inconveniences such as asthma, circulatory problems which caused her legs to swell, and headaches, some of which were legacies of her pregnancies. John, on his part, was not in good health, and had a hard time in properly dispatching the family businesses, including his professional commitments as a lawyer. By mid-1854, Susan was pregnant again with her third child, Mary Ashley, whose birth was due by the end of February, 1855. The prospect of being unable to travel farther than Danville for a year and perhaps longer plunged her into a deep crisis. Depression soon ensued and, between 1854 and 1856, especially when her husband was away, she would write desperate messages to her mother, such as: "I look for my husband tomorrow and will feel lost if he doesn't come for I am not only lonely but so much more timid than I need to be that I have scarcely slept since he left." On another instance she wrote: "in

[20] Susan P. Grigsby Correspondence, undated letters, 1854-55. Grigsby Family Papers. FHS.
[21] Susan P. Grigsby to her mother, Undated letters, 1854-1856. Grigsby Family Papers. FHS.
[22] Ibid.

addition to my solitary condition [I] have felt very unwell." After the birth of Mary Ashley she insisted: "I am lonely and unhappy."[23]

The diminished self-reliance of which Susan Grigsby was prey in 1855 was compounded by apprehensions about the well-being of her kin. That year an epidemic of cholera ravaged the Danville area, taking many human lives. In the severity of the hour, she would write her mother: "we are kept anxious & uneasy about the cholera, for there are so many deaths recurring in the neighborhood that we feel our time is yet to come."[24]

Although the Grigsbys were spared by cholera, Susan could not escape erysipelas, an infective, disagreeable skin disease which, years later, would also afflict her daughter Susie. "My dear mother," she wrote at some point, "I feel so bad from taking medicines in addition to my bodily sufferings, that I have not the heart to write to anyone except yourself." By then Susan was pregnant a fourth time, and her worries were amplified by the prospect of another long period of physical debilitation and confinement at a time when her body was already weakened by several ailments, including erysipelas. Under the circumstances, she could not hope to find temporary distraction from her many troubles and duties through the pursuit of self-gratifying activities such as the embellishment of her house and a modicum of social life would have offered. As her sense of isolation increased with the awareness of what her life would have been like in the following year or so, Susan's proverbial resourcefulness in positively reacting to adversities began to waver and slowly turned into passive acceptance of whatever life would bring. Extreme difficulty in fighting erysipelas probably played a major role in changing Susan P. Grigsby's outlook as she became persuaded that, after over two years of unsuccessful treatment, the disease was "so deeply rooted in [her] own system" that "no medicinal treatment could eradicate it."[25]

As the Grigsby household grew larger and larger, the problems generated by physical impairment and protracted periods of semi-invalidity increased exponentially, engendering a deep sense of helplessness and uselessness in Susan's mind. "I am a poor good for nothing creature," she complained, "at best a burden to all around me." In early 1856, her first two children were still small, the third was but a baby and, with a further one due soon, Susan felt at a loss in figuring out how she could run her household and estate. A privileged woman and the owner of many slaves,

[23] Susan P. Grigsby Correspondence, Undated letters, 1854-56. Grigsby Family Papers. FHS.
[24] Ibid.
[25] Ibid.

she could assign a number of them to domestic service, and to the care of her children. However, not all of them were suited for every task, and were not therefore interchangeable. Moreover, individual skills were not always matched by dependability, and Susan Grigsby attached much importance to that quality. In the effort to optimize her servants' performance, she therefore tried to train each of them in a single task—washing, cooking, sewing, and so on—according to their individual inclination.[26]

Being "methodical, thoughtful, kind, and very clean," Jennie was excellent in nursing the babies and taking care of the children in general. In Susan's opinion, also Mary could perform the same tasks rather satisfactorily, but only under constant guidance. So, she was perfect in that capacity only if sided by Jennie. Sarah, instead, was "too harum scarum" for Susan's patience which was, by her own admission, very limited. One time that Jennie was sick for several days, and unable to do any work, she [Sarah] "let every thing go to sack as that [one] morning not a set of clean clothes could be found for Alfred [her oldest son]." In other words, the temporary inability of a slave to perform the assigned task because of illness completely upset the routine in household management, and her attempt to apply the available ones to tasks they were unfamiliar with invariably resulted in disaster.[27]

It did not take long for Susan to realize that, because her almost chronic physical debilitation prevented her from effectively taking over the running of her household at critical times, she needed a white housekeeper to supervise and coordinate the work of the slave servants; someone whose authoritativeness rested on real knowledge of every department of housework. Securing one such person was however no mean feat. Although declaring themselves sincerely willing to learn, some of the applicants, mostly recent immigrants from Europe, were honest enough as to admit their utter inexperience. They had therefore to be discarded. Others were dropped on account of their bluntness in stating that they would not perform certain tasks. In a number of instances, applicants feigned competence and were therefore hired, but soon revealed themselves impostors and had to be dismissed. Even women who met Susan's requirements, and showed to have developed bonds of affection to the family, might leave without notice for a better employment.[28]

---

[26] Marli Weiner, *Mistresses and Slaves: Plantation Women in South Carolina, 1830-1880*. Chicago: University of Illinois Press, 1998), 8-13.

[27] Susan P. Grigsby to her mother. Undated letters, 1855-56. Grigsby Family Papers. FHS.

[28] Susan P. Grigsby Correspondence. Undated letters, 1856-58. Some of the Grigsby papers have been used by Stephanie Cole for the writing of her essay "A

Difficulties in securing the kind of help Susan was seeking were compounded by the rather isolated location of Traveller's Rest. Potential employees who lived in urban areas, and especially immigrant women, turned up their noses at the idea of removing to the countryside. One of them declared herself available for the job on condition that she be allowed to attend church service in Danville every Sunday. Even when temporarily satisfactory, Susan Grigsby's experiences with white domestic servants were, on the whole, disastrous. At some point in 1856 she was "so completely horrified at the confusion & filth" that she could not sit content and indulge the servants any longer. "I am very much wounded," she wrote her mother, "and forgot entirely when I insisted upon having Mrs. Queen stay with me."[29]

Although her first impulse was to revert to her slave servants exclusively, as she actually did for a brief time, her hopes to find the ideal white help did not completely subside. In 1857, when she had a fourth baby to nurse, Susan reiterated to her mother her ardent wish to have a white woman supervise her household. By that time, however, her exigencies had become even more diverse, if any possible. Her first two children, Alfred and Susie, who were eight and seven respectively, needed a governess but Mary Ashley and Virginia, aged four and three, still required a nurse. Moreover, Susan was pregnant again, and the newborn would have needed special care. She herself not only wanted companionship, but also somebody to relieve her of material duties during the several months she expected to be physically weakened and probably in pain. Under those circumstances, she not only simply looked for a jack of all tasks to supervise and eventually supplement the work of her domestic slaves; somebody who might even be relatively uneducated, provided she was competent and energetic. She definitely needed a woman of some education to instruct her older children, and with whom she could entertain polite and interesting conversation.

White Woman, of Middle Age, Would Be preferred: Children's Nurses in the Old South," in Susanna Delfino and Michele Gillespie, eds., *Neither Lady Nor Slave: Working Women of the Old South* (Chapel Hill, NC: University of North Carolina press, 2002) 75-101. See also Faye Dudden, *Serving Women: Household Service in Nineteenth Century America* (Middletown, CT: Wesleyan University Press, 1985), 35-65; Margaret Lynch-Brennan, *The Irish Bridget: Irish Immigrant Women in Domestic Service in America, 1840-1939* (Syracuse, N.Y.: Syracuse University Press, 2009), 65-73.

[29] Susan P. Grigsby Correspondence. Undated letters, probably 1857. Grigsby Family Papers. FHS.

When Jane Drummond arrived, in early 1859, Susan had just given birth to Hart, her fifth child. Little is known about this woman, who was about seven years older than her. A Jamaican by birth, she had moved to the States with her parents some time earlier, and settled in Trenton, New Jersey. Although the Drummonds may have previously enjoyed financial comfort, as suggested by the fact that Jane had received an education, their circumstances in the United States seem to have been rather modest as to prompt Jane to find employment as a governess and lady companion. The two women liked each other immediately, and established a wonderful, mutually satisfactory relationship. With Jane's arrival everything seemed to go better in the Grigsby household, and Susan looked more serene and optimistic than she had been for a long time. The very special way, sweet and gentle, with which she related to the children soon earned "Drummy"—as they familiarly addressed her—their unconditional affection. She schooled Alfred and Susie, played with Mary and Virginia, lulled little Hart, assisted and entertained Susan without ever losing touch with the general affairs of the household. Convalescence after Hart's birth was expectedly long and painful, complicated as it was by chronic health problems. At such a delicate time in her life, Susan's preoccupations were compounded by news of her mother's critical health condition due to a heart disease, probably angina. Virginia's death, in early May 1859, literally devastated Susan, who had always adored her mother and held her an irreplaceable confident and advisor throughout her life. In all likelihood, she would not have been able to get over the trials she endured in 1859 without Drummond's moral and material support.[30]

Susan's mother had for some time been affected by severe nervous disturbances, the result of decades of physical and mental wear. The untimely loss of her first husband and their fourth child, the heavy commitments connected with the running of the family businesses, and the death of her two sons by Alfred had undermined her nervous system over time. Her second marriage had brought more challenges to her: three close pregnancies, the handling of a large family which included her husband's eight children, the death of one of her three children by Robert, and the stormy relationship with him, which almost ended with divorce, had put so much strain on her body and mind that she had become increasingly

[30] Susan Hart Shelby Fishback to Susan Grigsby, August 4, 1859; John Grigsby to wife Susan, August 24, 1859; Jane Drummond to Susan Grigsby, October 31, 1859. Grigsby Family Papers. FHS.

acrimonious, even hysterical. Finally, she had developed a heart disease, perhaps angina, which caused her much physical suffering.[31]

With her mother's demise, Susan lost her confident and the last member of her family of origin. Her only consolation was now having the friendship and companionship of Jane Drummond. Life circumstances, however, would soon deprive her also of this last mooring. In 1860, Drummond was suddenly recalled home by news of her father's severe illness. She left with the promise to return to Kentucky as soon as possible but she could not, either because of further impediments created by her mother's and other old relatives' precarious health conditions and of intervening difficulties connected with the outbreak of the Civil War. Drummond was not there to assist and support Susan Grigsby through the major ordeals she had to cope with between 1860 and 1862: the birth of Lilie Shelby and the death of five of her children, two of whom were but infants, while her husband was away at war, fighting on the Confederate side.[32]

The tragic death of so many of her children might have easily driven Susan insane for the rest of her life. Yet, having far trespassed the threshold of endurance of sorrow and grief that a human being can possibly bear, the abysmal despair in which she sank after those tremendous losses almost petrified her. She looked for comfort in prayer, Christianly bowing to the will of God. Between late 1862 and early 1863, Susan was seriously determined to cross the confederate line with some servants and her two surviving children, Virginia and Hart, and look for her husband. To this effect, she secured a pass from the federal military authorities in her area, and made a last effort to convince Jane Drummond to join the party. Although regretfully, she waived the invitation on account of her poor financial resources that, as she claimed, not only compelled her to work for a living, but were anyway insufficient to finance a journey to Kentucky. Dissuaded by her dearest relatives, Susan never undertook that perilous journey down south.[33]

---

[31] Robert J. Breckinridge Memorandum, September 20, 1856. Robert J. Breckinridge Papers. Library of Congress, Manuscript Division. Susan P. Grigsby to "Dearest Aunt," April 3, 1859. Grigsby Family Papers. FHS.

[32] W. H. Perrin, et al., *Kentucky: A History of the State* (Louisville, KY: F. A. Battey Co., 1887), 779.

[33] Jane Drummond to Susan Grigsby, November 5, 1862; Susan H. Fishbach to Susan P. Grigsby, November 2 1862, January 3 1863; Letitia Wallace to Susan Grigsby, 1862, and undated correspondence, 1862-63. Grigsby Family Papers. FHS.

At the end of the conflict, John Grigsby returned home to embrace a woman who was so different from the one he had left three years earlier. Twelve years of married life during which she had borne seven children, and the many ordeals she had gone through during the Civil War had produced incurable scars in Susan's body and psyche as well. The thirty five-year-old woman he had before his eyes in 1865 was no longer the good-looking, cheerful young lady he had married fifteen years earlier. Her beauty most probably faded, her strength of purpose severely weakened, Susan could not hide from her husband that she felt as if she were a century old. On the other hand, John's already delicate health had been much proven by the wartime rigors. Yet, life must go on, and the two of them found in mutual love the resource to reinvent the future and rebuild their fortunes on the ashes of a bygone era. They took the challenge in the awareness that nothing was going to be the same as before. Susan's once remarkable wealth was far reduced by the loss of her slaves, and John's financial position, which had never been florid, was even more fragile than it had been before the war. To testify to their confidence in a new departure, they had two more children, both girls, and resumed their time-old, high maintenance lifestyle, buying expensive tableware and foodstuffs.[34]

The post-war years were however tough enough as to force the Grigsbys to scale down their expectations. As a matter of fact, they had to increasingly erode their assets to stay afloat and, when John died in 1877, Susan found herself deeply indebted. A woman of forty-six, with a weaker and weaker network of trustworthy relatives to rely on, either because some of them had passed away and the remaining ones were too old and impoverished to assist her, Susan Grigsby was conscious that her resources were too scant to allow her to weather alone the challenges of the post-Reconstruction era. After John's death, in early 1877, she had no alternativc to honor his liabilities but to surrender Traveller's Rest to her major creditor: Mrs. Hart, the widow of her beloved uncle "Bill."[35]

Thereafter, Susan Grigsby became increasingly estranged from the small world in which she had been born and had lived most of her life. As her personal attachments became fewer and fewer, and her financial difficulties more and more stringent, she felt that there was no place anymore for her among the society where she had long been looked at with consideration and respect as a member of the prestigious Shelby

[34] Walton and Brother to Susan P. Grigsby, December 4 1868; D. H. Cowan to Susan P. Grigsby,September 20, 1869. Grigsby Family Papers. FHS.
[35] Biographical Sketch of John Warren Grigsby; J. W. Stevenson to John Cowan, March 26, 1877. Grigsby Family Papers. FHS.

family. Pressed by major financial difficulties she was unable to cope with, Susan matured the conviction that times were ripe for a major change in perspective, and that she should adapt to the new reality of a woman who needed a gainful employment to support herself and her family.

In 1883, thanks to the good offices of her first cousin, Louisiana senator Randall Lee Gibson, Susan was able to secure employment for herself and her daughter Virginia in the federal Land Office and the Post Office, respectively.[36] By the time she moved her family to D.C., Susan was fifty-three, her oldest child, Virginia Shelby, was twenty-seven, Hart Preston twenty-three, and the two younger ones, Louisiana and Susanna, still adolescents. Her courageous resolve to relocate in the national capital did not simply stem from her pressing need to make ends meet, but also from her desire to provide her offspring with the necessary introductions they could seize to build their own future in an urban area of the east coast where opportunities did not lack.[37]

Once the mistress of a large plantation, and therefore vowed to an existence of hard work and self-sacrifice in behalf of her household and estate without receiving any recognition—either private or public—for her exertions, Susan was catapulted into a world in which women could command social respect and earn personal independence through honest, remunerated work.[38]

The Civil War experience had infused in her, as in many other women of her generation, a new sense of self-reliance and a desire for autonomy which was per se revolutionary, for it implied the abandonment of traditional notions of correct behavior upper class females were expected to comply with, including the inappropriateness of plying a gainful occupation. The conflict had indeed transformed an aristocratic southern lady like Susan Shelby Grigsby into a bourgeois woman whose priorities were no longer determined by the idolization of family lineage and prestige to the point of maintaining a façade of gentility at any cost, but by practical decisions aimed at procuring a comfortable living and some financial security to herself and her offspring. In this new perspective,

---

[36] Randall L. Gibson to Susan Grigsby, 1883. Grigsby Family Papers. FHS.

[37] Sarah G. Humphreys to Susan Grigsby, May 26 1883. Grigsby Family Papers, FHS; Mary McBride and Ann McLaurin, "Sarah G. Humphreys: Antebellum Belle to Equal Rights Activist, 1830-1907," *Filson Club History Quarterly* 65 (1991), 244-45.

[38] Susanna Delfino and Michele Gillespie. *Neither Lady nor Slave: Working Women of the Old South* (Columbia, MO: University of Missouri Press, 2002), introduction.

understandings of family respectability and pride in its illustrious origins took on a new meaning which was not at odds with self-support through paid work.

* * *

The sufferings Susan Grigsby had endured throughout her life—the untimely loss of her father, little sister, her two brothers, five of her children, and the death of her dear mother and husband—had produced incurable scars in her mind and soul. Although still in her early fifties, when she moved to D.C. Susan felt that an important part of herself had been buried with them. Her body, too, carried the marks of the many diseases and ailing conditions that had maimed it over time. Painful as that all had been, it was past, and to the past she consigned the memory of both the good and bad times she had lived as the scion of a prominent southern family between the antebellum and Civil War eras. The demise of the Old South had not found her unprepared to meet the new challenges. Yet, for some time thereafter, she had clung to old ideas of aristocratic gentility in the handling of the family businesses and financial matters. Only after John's death did she realize that the key words of the new times were "calculation" and "profit," in utter disregard of the people's individual sensibilities and difficulties. After losing her beloved Traveller's Rest because of her inability to honor the payments of its mortgage, Susan Grigsby fully understood the assumptions underlying interpersonal relations and business transactions in post-Civil War America. Her undoubtedly momentous decision to relocate her family to Washington, D.C., would have helped her get over the many worries and mourning that had accompanied her life in the olden era. Suspended between past and future, Susan Grigsby embraced the latter and cast her and her children's fortunes with the opportunities purported by the new times.

With hindsight, it is interesting to compare Susan Grigsby's reaction to her personal tragedies and challenges with those faced by her mother. Although a strong-willed and enterprising woman, Virginia Hart (Shelby) Breckinridge was never able to free herself from the shackles of a male-dominated southern culture that confined women to an officially gregarious role, and made them captives to social conventions that denied them public recognition of their fundamental agency in the running of their families' businesses. With no hope of ever being able to emancipate themselves from the social prescriptions that required them to live in the shadow of men as wives, mothers, and alter egos of their husbands, many of them slowly but inexorably developed nervous disturbances:

depression, anxiety, a sense of persecution, and even schizophrenia. Such psychical conditions were enhanced by constant fear that diseases of various descriptions might put at risk their own lives and those of their children as well. And when life repeatedly presented them with major trials such as the death of a child or other kin, even the most combative among those women might lose control of their emotions, and become fatalistic. This is what happened to Susan's mother, Virginia H. Shelby Breckinridge, whose initial energy, vitality, and purposefulness were progressively weakened by the combined effect of the strain resulting from her being a woman entrepreneur in a male-dominated society, and the devastations that the loss of her first husband and four of her children had produced on her psyche. Although Susan shared with her mother many similar experiences, and despite the fact that she was much less psychologically independent and strong-willed than Virginia, the improvements in the condition of women purported by the rebirth of America after the demise of the Old South enabled her to see a feeble light at the end of the tunnel in which she was advancing deeper and deeper, and infused in her a desire for survival that her mother had instead been denied.

Toward the end of the 1880s, Susan P. Grigsby was "almost worn out into life and its disappointments" and confessed to dear cousin Sarah: "In my intensely nervous condition—my precious children sometimes think me deranged—and indeed they are not far mistaken…" Feeling that her work in this world was almost done, she only longed to "be steered across the Lilley-lined shore of the River of rest!" She died of pneumonia in Washington, D.C., on November 7, 1891, at the age of sixty-one. Had her husband still been alive, the previous day they would have celebrated their forty-first wedding anniversary. But dear John was no longer with her, and she may have felt that, perhaps, it was high time for her to join him. So she did.[39]

Works Cited

Manuscript sources

Filson Historical Society, Louisville, Kentucky:
Carter, Horace, Letters 1835-1839.
Grigsby Family, Papers 1818-1891.
Hegewald, Mina Conrad, Louisville Notes.

---

[39] "Death of Mrs. Susan P. Grigsby," typescript, 1891, Grigsby Family Papers.

Irwin, John, Letters 1832-1840.
Jefferson, John, Diary 1857-1860.
Library of Congress, Manuscript Division, Washington, D.C.: Breckinridge Family, Robert J. Breckinridge, Papers 1837-1856.
Special Collections, University of Kentucky, Lexington: Jones, John W., Papers 1841-1862.
Kentucky Department of Libraries and Archives: Fayette County, Marriage Records, 1850.

Historical literature

Clinton, Catherine. *Plantation Mistress: Woman's World in the Old South.* New York: Pantheon, 1982.
—. *Tara Revisited: Women, War, & the Plantation Legend.* New York: Abbeville Press, 1995.
Cole, Stephanie. "A White Woman, of Middle Age, Would Be Preferred: Children's Nurses in the Old South." Delfino and Gillespie, 75-101.
Coryell, Janet, et al. *Negotiating the Boundaries of Southern Womanhood: Dealing with the Powers that Be.* Columbia, MO: University of Missouri Press, 2000.
Delfino, Susanna and Michele Gillespie, eds. *Neither Lady nor Slave: Working Women of the Old South.* Columbia, MO: University of Missouri Press, 2002.
Dudden, Faye, *Serving Women: Household Service in Nineteenth Century America.* Middletown, CT: Wesleyan University Press, 1985.
Fox-Genovese, Elizabeth. *Within the Plantation Household: Black and White Women of the Old South.* Chapel Hill, NC: University of North Carolina Press, 1988.
Fought, Leigh. *Southern Womanhood and Slavery: A Biography of Louisa S. McCord, 1810-1879.* Columbia, MO: University of Missouri Press, 2003.
Fredrickson, Dorman. *The Prestons of Smithfield and Greenfield in Virginia.* Louisville, KY: Filson Club Publications, 2nd ser., n. 3, 1982.
Henderson, Archibald. "Isaac Shelby: Revolutionary Patriot and Border Hero." *The North Carolina Booklet* 16 (1917).
Klotter, James C. *The Breckinridges of Kentucky, 1760-1981.* Lexington, KY: The University Press of Kentucky, 1981.
Leavitt, Judith W. *Brought to Bed: Childbearing in America, 1750-1950.* New York: Oxford University Press, 1986.

Lynch-Brennan, Margaret. *The Irish Bridget: Irish Immigrant Women in Domestic Service in America, 1840-1939*. Syracuse, N.Y.: Syracuse University Press, 2009.

McBride, Mary and Ann McLaurin. "Sarah G. Humphreys: Antebellum Belle to Equal Rights Activist, 1830-1907." *Filson Club History Quarterly* 65 (1991): 231-51.

Perrin, W. H. et al. *Kentucky: A History of the State*. Louisville, KY: F. A. Battey Co., 1887.

Scott, Anne Firor. *The Southern Lady: From Pedestal to Politics, 1830-1930*. Chicago: University of Chicago Press, 1970.

Weiner, Marli. *Mistresses and Slaves: Plantation Women in South Carolina, 1830-1880*. Chicago: University of Illinois Press, 1998.

Wertz, Richard W. and Dorothy Wertz. *Living-In: A History of Childbirth in America*. New York: Free Press, 1977.

CHAPTER SEVEN

ILLNESS AS METAPHOR IN THE SOUTH: LILLIAN SMITH'S DIAGNOSIS OF A SCHIZOPHRENIC CULTURE AND A METASTASIZED SOCIAL BODY*

CONSTANTE GONZÁLEZ GROBA

> Racism is a disease, a historical ill, a disorder of the historical self, and it reflects the fullness of that self even as it reveals its inadequacies. For wherever the sense of individual self is most highly developed and at the same time most dynamically torn—and where is this more true than in the West, and most of all, in America?—racism is there most instilled into the fabric of culture.[1]

Illness has always been a major political tool in the construction of the racial other. Kathryn Stockett's novel *The Help* (2009), set in the early 1960s, provides us with some clear examples of the kind of tools that white southern women used against African Americans in the days of segregation in Jackson, Mississippi. Freudians have always defined neurotic behavior as defensive and built on repressions and projections.[2] The most neurotic character in *The Help* is Hilly Holbrook, who refers to African Americans as "those *other* people."[3] Like most of the other white women in the novel, Hilly nourishes her body with food prepared by black maids, while emotionally she is dependent on an invigorating diet of the

* The research leading to the publication of this essay was financed by the Spanish Ministry of Economy and Competitiveness (Project FFI2010-17061).

[1] Joel Kovel, *White Racism: A Phychohistory* (London: Free Association Books, 1988), 232.

[2] Earl E. Thorpe, *The Old South: A Phychohistory* (Durham, N. C.: Seeman Printery, 1972), 63.

[3] Kathryn Stockett, *The Help* (London: Penguin Books, 2010), 205.

dogma of white supremacy, a doctrine which renders black people as mere things, abstract equivalents of bodily filth. Hilly is obsessed with the idea that whites must protect themselves from the diseases of black people, as seen in the note that she gives to her friend Skeeter to publish in the Newsletter of the Junior League of Jackson:

> *Hilly Holbrook introduces the Home Help Sanitation Initiative. A disease preventative measure. Low-cost bathroom installation in your garage or shed, for homes without such an important fixture.*
> *Ladies, did you know that:*
> - *99% of all colored diseases are carried in the urine*
> - *Whites can become permanently disabled by nearly all of these diseases because we lack immunities coloreds carry in their darker pigmentation*
> - *Some germs carried by whites can also be harmful to coloreds too*
>
> *Protect yourself. Protect your children. Protect your help.*
> *From the Holbrooks, we say, You're welcome!*[4]

Stockett's novel exposes the need that whites had for intimate but unequal relations with blacks. Black maids cook and clean for whites and nurse their children, but they cannot eat at the same table or use the same bathrooms. In her autobiography *The Making of a Southerner* (1946) the progressive white southerner Katharine Du Pre Lumpkin refers to the importance in her racial conversion of "eating with Negroes" for the first time. Because it granted blacks the privilege of "social equality," Lumpkin notes that "In the whole roster of Southern taboos it was nearly the most sacred. It was a grievous Southern sin for which were allowed no mitigating circumstances."[5] Often characterized by their simplistic reduction of the human world to the influences of the unconscious, Freudian interpretations argue that the intensity of the negation or rejection of African Americans is manifested in their identification with faeces and other excretions of the body, with everything that is low-down and dirty, and which has to be excreted or "segregated" from the social body. Joel Kovel, for instance, argues: "The nuclear experience of the aversive racist is a sense of disgust about the body of the black person based upon a very primitive fantasy: that it contains an essence—dirt—that smells and may rub off onto the body of the racist. Hence the need for distance and the prohibition against touching."[6]

---

[4] Stockett, *The Help*, 158.
[5] Katharine Du Pre Lumpkin, *The Making of a Southerner* (Athens: The University of Georgia Press, 1991), 206.
[6] Kovel, *White Racism*, 84.

The use of the threat of uncleanness and disease as a political tool to exclude African Americans has a long tradition in the American South. The conception of blacks as carriers of disease goes back to the very beginning of slavery, when whites tried to reconcile their racist practices with their professed Christianity by considering blacks as biologically inferior, as little more than animals with no soul. The Civil War years brought with them a proliferation of racist theories. One famous advocate of the racial status quo was the New York physician Dr. J. H. Van Evrie, whose aim was to persuade white working men that African Americans were biologically and permanently inferior and that slavery should not be disturbed. On the eve of the Civil War, in his book titled *Negroes and Negro "Slavery:" The First an Inferior Race: The Latter Its Normal Condition* (1861), this self-proclaimed scientist contended that slavery was the "normal condition" of African Americans, and that "the social order of the South" encouraged the "civilization, progress, and general welfare of both races."[7] He assured racists that the parental affections of black people were very weak and that "the strongest affection" a slave "is capable of feeling is love for his master."[8] Free blacks were unnatural and "destined to extinction" in the American nation.[9] In a previous shorter version of *Negroes and Negro "Slavery,"* subtitled *Introductory Number: Causes of the Popular Delusion on the Subject* (1853), he had already asserted that the African American "is not a black white man, or a man merely with a black skin, but a DIFFERENT AND INFERIOR SPECIES OF MAN,"[10] and that his brain is much smaller than that of Caucasians and thus "its acquisition of knowledge is limited to a single generation, and incapable of transmitting this to subsequent ones."[11] He warned that "intermingling the blood of races essentially different" would lead to "social suicide."[12]

After slavery was abolished, white southerners became even more obsessed with asserting their superiority over African Americans, and all kinds of medical and scientific theories were used to justify the need for segregation, for maintaining the "purity" of the South's ethnic and social body. Part of the myth of the Lost Cause was the idea that African

---

[7] J. H. Van Evrie, *Negroes and Negro "Slavery:" The First, an Inferior Race: The Latter Its Normal Condition* (New York: Van Evrie, Horton & Co., 1861), 201.

[8] Ibid., 191.

[9] Ibid., 309.

[10] J. H. Van Evrie, *Negroes and Negro "Slavery;" The First, an Inferior Race—The Latter Its Normal Condition. Introductory Number: Causes of Popular Delusion on the Subject* (Baltimore: John D. Toy, 1853), 2.

[11] Ibid., 29.

[12] Ibid., 18.

Americans actually suffered from their freedom and were as a result afflicted by numerous physical and mental diseases. To justify slavery and the subjugation of blacks that followed Reconstruction, disease was made into a political and social tool to instil fear. Disease and uncleanness became foreign, non-white. The Lost Cause advocate Myrta Lockett Avary claimed in her book *Dixie after the War* (1906):

> After freedom, they [blacks] began to die of pulmonary complaints. There were frequent epidemics of typhoid fever, quarters not being well kept. 'The race is dying out,' said prophets. Negroes began to grow mad. An insane negro was rarely heard of during slavery. Regular hours, regular work, chiefly out of doors, sobriety, freedom from care and responsibility had kept the negro singularly exempt from insanity and various other afflictions that curse the white. Big lunatic asylums established for negroes soon after the war and their continual enlargement tell their own story.[13]

Avary added to her analysis the claim that child abuse and syphilis were also rampant within the black community. As Catherine Clinton says, Avary, like others of her circle, "manifested extreme anxiety over the questions of flesh, blood, and interracial sex that raged during this tumultuous period, as they had for generations."[14]

In the early 1890s Dr. Eugene Rollin Corson, a well-known physician from Savannah, gave a paper on "The Vital Equation of the Colored Race and Its Future in the United States." He attributed the high mortality rate of blacks not to environmental conditions or social exclusion, but to the end of the "old regime [of slavery], where they were well cared for." He argued that the younger generations of blacks, deprived from birth of the paternalistic protection of slavery, were liable to be even more widely affected by a variety of diseases which supposedly hit blacks harder than whites. The excessively high rate of black mortality simply confirmed "the teachings of ethnology and biology" about the anatomical and physical inferiority of African Americans. And because they did not have the intelligence to care for themselves, they rapidly reverted to savagery once freed from the control of slave owners. Dr. Corson's final verdict was that the black race would ultimately disappear, a victim of "the struggle for existence against a superior race."[15]

---

[13] Myrta Lockett Avary, *Dixie after the War* (New York: Doubleday, Page & Company, 1906), 196.

[14] Catherine Clinton, *Tara Revisited: Women, War, & the Plantation Legend* (New York: Abbeville Press, 1995), 179.

[15] Quoted in George M. Fredrickson, *The Black Image in the White Mind* (New York: Harper Torchbooks, 1971), 248.

In 1896 the German-born insurance statistician Frederick L. Hoffman published the book *Race Traits and Tendencies of the American Negro*, described by George M. Fredrickson as "the most influential discussion of the race question to appear in the late nineteenth century."[16] The book helped to convince most white insurance companies that they should not give cover to blacks, since being a member of this racial group brought with it an unacceptable risk. In a letter to Edward Eggleston (Aug. 5, 1910), a racial propagandist from Virginia, Hoffman wrote that, partly as a result of his research, "our company [the Prudential] has not for a number of years insured Negroes except in cases where we were compelled to do so in compliance with the Law."[17] Hoffman did not share the worries of those who feared that the black population could come to outnumber the whites. He contended, rather, that the black mortality rate had increased dramatically since emancipation, at which time the black population had been in excellent physical condition.

Most of the diseases of African Americans were not due to environmental conditions but to racial characteristics. Some were the result of the "inferior organisms and constitutional weakness"[18] of African Americans and others originated from "the fact of an immense amount of immorality which is a race trait, and of which scrofula, syphilis, and even consumption are the inevitable consequences."[19] The prediction was that all these characteristics and tendencies would in the end cause the extinction of the black race. The belief of Hoffman and many other racists of the period was that the black race was so imperfect that neither religion nor education could contribute to its improvement and that its poverty was not due to discrimination but was "the natural and inevitable result of crime and immorality"[20] which they considered to be innate traits of black people.

Lillian Smith (1897-1966) was one of the very few white southerners of her time to denounce racial segregation, which she opposed in practically all her fiction, articles, speeches and newspaper work. Just as the northern abolitionists and even some southern emancipators like Thomas Jefferson had identified slavery itself as the disease, as a cancer on the body politic of the South, Smith turned the racist argument around and diagnosed the segregated South as a pathological society and explained how segregation made southerners psychologically sick. Influenced by her

---

[16] George M. Fredrickson, *The Black Image in the White Mind*, 249.
[17] Quoted in Fredrickson, *The Black Image*, 250n36.
[18] Frederick L Hoffman, *Race Traits and Tendencies of the American Negro* (New York: The Macmillan Company, 1896), 66.
[19] Ibid., 95.
[20] Ibid., 241.

reading of Freudian psychology, she paid attention to the individual not only as a social being, but also as existing in a body which translates sensory impressions into symptoms, into marks in what Freudians call the "subconscious." For Freudians to talk about the body is to talk about sexuality, about prohibitions, about relations within the family. In her autobiographical book *Killers of the Dream* (1949, revised 1961), Smith refers to the enforced rituals of white supremacy which make white children into automatons, and she notes: "These ceremonials in honor of white supremacy, performed from babyhood, slip from the conscious mind down deep into muscles and glands and become difficult to tear out."[21] Political power penetrates the bodies and haunts the childhood of white children. In the culture of segregation in which Lillian Smith was raised, the body itself became a site of political contention. Segregation is a system in which bodies are not allowed to be whole or to extend naturally in space, and their impenetrability and sanctity are always vulnerable, carrying sexual and racial marks.

Southern children do not grow up healthy and free. On the contrary, Smith notes, "we are stunted and warped and in our lifetime cannot grow straight again any more than can a tree, put in a steel-like twisting frame when young, grow tall and straight when the frame is torn away at maturity."[22] To be a southerner is to be the victim of a social system that is an instrument of torture, making one socially and psychically deformed. And this torture and deformity affect children of both races: "I began to understand slowly at first but more clearly as the years passed, that the warped, distorted frame we have put around every Negro child from birth is around every white child also. Each is on a different side of the frame but each is pinioned there. And I knew that what cruelly shapes and cripples the personality of one is as cruelly shaping and crippling the personality of the other."[23] With her insistence that segregation irreparably damages whites as well as blacks, Smith seems in some way to anticipate Toni Morrison's argument in *Playing in the Dark* that America cannot do without its African presence, that Africanism is the vehicle through which the American defines his self, that whiteness depends on blackness to define as well as to enhance itself. As Morrison maintains, "images of blackness can be evil *and* protective, rebellious *and* forgiving, fearful *and* desirable—all of the self-contradictory features of the self. Whiteness, alone, is mute, meaningless, unfathomable, pointless, frozen, veiled,

---

[21] Lillian Smith, *Killers of the Dream*, revised edition (New York: Norton, 2004), 96.

[22] Ibid., 39.

[23] Ibid., 39.

curtained, dreaded, senseless, implacable. Or so our writers seem to say."[24] Smith warns her fellow white southerners that by obsessively emphasizing their whiteness to the total exclusion of blackness, "we have shut ourselves away from the good, the creative, the human in life."[25]

Lillian Smith stressed the idea that the private and the social body came together, and was the writer who most explicitly described the connections between racial and sexual segregation, which to her were powerful emblems of the cultural schizophrenia of southern society. In one famous passage she establishes a metaphorical parallel between the segregated parts of the white female child's body and the segregated spaces of southern towns, and simultaneously points to the relations between the legacy of racial segregation and that of Victorian sexual repression. For a white southern child to explore blackness entailed as great a risk as exploring one's own body:

> By the time we were five years old we had learned, without hearing the words, that masturbation is wrong and segregation is right, and each had become a dread taboo that must never be broken, for we believed God, whom we feared and tried desperately to love, had made the rules concerning not only Him and our parents, but our bodies and Negroes. Therefore when we as small children crept over the race line and ate and played with Negroes or broke other segregation customs known to us, we felt the same dread fear of consequences, the same overwhelming guilt we felt when we crept over the sex line and played with our body.[26]

The God that sanctions segregation and instils in whites a fear of dark people is the same God that instils in the faithful a fear of the creative powers of their own bodies. Sexuality is dark and should be repressed with the same vehemence as blacks. In fact, at the core of the doctrine inculcated into southern children is the principle that "Not only Negroes but everything dark, dangerous, evil must be pushed to the rim of one's life."[27] Thus the white southerner is turned into a broken, diminihed being by his own culture, one that suppresses not only the humanity of blacks but also the creative and precious darkness in himself. For Smith, then, integration was more than a strategy to improve race relations; it was the effort to restore the wholeness of the individual and to stop the

---

[24] Toni Morrison, *Playing in the Dark: Whiteness and the Literary Imagination* (New York: Vintage, 1993), 59.

[25] Lillian Smith, "Growing into Freedom," *Common Ground* 4, no.1 (Autumn 1943): 51.

[26] Lillian Smith, *Killers of the Dream*, 83-84.

[27] Ibid., 90.

compartmentalization of a culture characterized by blocked doors preventing the free flow of vital energies. She insistently voiced her concern about what segregation does to white children, which is in some ways a sort of reflection of that done to black children, as if both are marked by the same deprivation of healthy emotional growth in a culture of segregation. Firmly convinced of the interdependence of human beings, she could see no hope of a solution until whites acknowledged the blackness in themselves.

Lillian Smith was convinced that the huge advances in modern psychology and psychiatry could play a vital part in the transformation of cultures and societies. She actually made psychiatry into a new religion, in that the southern church had deviated from true Christianity. In "Humans in Bondage," an article from 1944, she wrote: "As for love … once preachers preached about it, and then lost their own belief in its magic. But psychiatrists have rediscovered it. They are telling us that love is powerful medicine in emotional illness, as specific for many mental 'infections' as penicillin for physical ailments. Perhaps the church will take courage from science and once more declare its faith in the love of God and man."[28] Smith always studied the workings of racism in terms of psychological illness and its consequent social harms.

Smith considered southern culture as schizophrenic and emphasized the parallel between racism splitting the world and its splitting of the racist's personality. For her the schizophrenic was the person who "has completely lost his ability to love and to make human identifications," and she was convinced that "when we reserve this humanity of ours, this precious quality of love, of tenderness, and of imaginative identification, for only people of our skin color […] we have split our lives in a way shockingly akin to those sick people whom we call schizophrenics."[29] A seminal idea in the work of Smith is Mahatma Gandhi's view that colonial situations equally diminish and split the personalities of the victims and the victimizers.[30] In a letter to Guy B. Johnson, executive director of the

---

[28] Lillian Smith, "Humans in Bondage," *The Winner Names the Age: A Collection of Writings by Lillian Smith*, ed. Michelle Cliff (New York: Norton, 1978), 54.

[29] Ibid., 38.

[30] Lillian Smith's residence in China as a music teacher in a Methodist music school, from 1923 to 1925, was crucial for her intellectual development and gave a specific international dimension to her thinking about the modern world. In her biography of Smith, Anne Loveland contends: "Her political consciousness was awakened for the first time as she observed the operation of European colonialism and the aftermath of the Chinese Revolution of 1911 and 1912 and as she heard and read about Mahatma Gandhi's fight for Indian independence." See Anne C.

Southern Regional Council, she described segregation as "spiritual lynching" and maintained that "the lynched and the lynchers are our own people, our own selves."[31] Smith denounced the severe harm that the practice of segregation, "a form of cultural schizophrenia, bearing a curious resemblance to the schizophrenia of individual personality,"[32] does to every southern child, both black and white, marked by the same deprivation of healthy emotional growth in a culture of segregation: "No colored child in our South is being given today what his personality needs in order to grow and mature richly and fully. No white child, under the segregation pattern, can be free of arrogance and hardness of heart, and blindness to human need—and hence no white child can grow freely and creatively under the crippling frame of segregation."[33] Smith could hardly be more precise in her description of the connection between racial segregation and psychological fracture, of the immense spiritual damage of an illusory racial identity.

It was her conviction that the culture of segregation split the mind of southerners that impelled Smith to write *Killers of the Dream*, to show that for her, segregation was not just racial but a psychologically harming alienation from reality, and to persuade fellow southerners "that [they could] no longer lean on walls that do not exist," that they should "accept [themselves] and all the earth's people as human beings" so that they could make "a world of open spaces with no walls in minds or between nations to throw their shadows across [their] children's lives."[34] For the world to change, each individual should change himself, and for the change to happen it was indispensable to pull down the walls that today still shape our thinking and our culture, walls that in the South, according to Smith, turned people's minds "into segregated compartments," so much so that southerners could "believe simultaneously in brotherhood and racial discrimination."[35] Smith defined racial discrimination as "a strong

---

Loveland, *Lillian Smith: A Southerner Confronting the South* (Baton Rouge: Louisiana State University Press, 1986), 12.

[31] Lillian Smith, Letter of June 12, 1944 to Guy B. Johnson, executive director of the SRC, *How Am I to Be Heard? Letters of Lillian Smith*, ed. Margaret Rose Gladney (Chapel Hill: University of North Carolina Press, 1993), 87.

[32] Ibid., 86.

[33] Ibid., 87.

[34] Lillian Smith, Letter of February 18, 1950, to unknown recipient, *How Am I to Be Heard?*, 132.

[35] Lillian Smith, "The Moral and Political Significance of the Students' Non-Violent Protests," *The Winner Names the Age*, 95.

wall behind which weak egos have hidden for a long time."[36] Segregation, with its psychologically comforting division into white and black, pure and impure, is a psychological defense mechanism. Mental walls provide a false sense of security and satisfy misguided mental needs; they do not protect us as much from dangerous others but from our own anxieties and fears; they are built more for those who live inside than for those outside. When we build a wall, we are really building a state of mind, a source of mental ease, a protection against the anarchic and the unknown in ourselves. In this sense, a wall is an implicit admission of vulnerability on the part of what Smith terms "weak egos." According to Costica Bradatan, "Once the wall has been erected, it acquires a life of its own and structures people's lives according to its own rules. It gives them meaning and a sense of direction."[37] This is precisely the point that Lillian Smith makes when she argues that "many southerners have used the walls of segregation so long to lean on psychologically that they will find it very hard to stand on their own feet as human beings, when the walls go," with the risk of collapse into mental illness. She adds that "It is going to be hard for every one of us, no matter how stable and objective, to create within our own minds the new image of ourselves as mature human beings"[38] independently of our skin color.

Lillian Smith made ample use of the metaphor of the fortified old house of southern tradition, a metaphor which echoes another, that of the walls which structure people's lives according to their own rules and give them meaning. In her writings she tried to expose and to heal the cracks that were spreading across the walls of that house. Having experienced in herself the closing of doors that alienates the self from reality, she strove to find ways to push them open. Such an opening could take place only after a process of painful self-scrutiny leading to the understanding of the internal segregation of the individual, which itself served to maintain the outward segregation of socicty. *Killers of the Dream* is in essence an invitation for the reader to accompany her in this opening of doors that will allow "glimpses of the world beyond, of that bright thing we call 'reality.'"[39] For Smith integration was not just a strategy to improve race relations but also the effort to restore the wholeness of the individual and

---

[36] Lillian Smith, "Ten Years from Today," *The Winner Names the Age*, 62.
[37] Costica Bradatan, "Scaling the 'Wall in the Head,'" *New York Times* Nov. 27, 2011. http://opinionator.blogs.nytimes.com/2011/11/27/scaling-the-wall-in-the-head/?nl=todayshe
[38] Lillian Smith, "Ten Years from Today," *The Winner Names the Age*, 63.
[39] Lillian Smith, *Killers of the Dream*, 30.

stop the compartmentalization of a culture characterized by blocked doors preventing the free flow of ideas and vital energies.

Firmly convinced that a racist society is pathological, Lillian Smith did not merely analyze the spiritual sickness of the South from the perspective of Freudianism and Christian humanism. She had the firm conviction that direct socio-political action is necessary if we want to change a social situation. Psychoanalysis alone can do very little to stop oppression or irrational fears if we do not change the status of the victims, if we do not change the pathogenic context. She became a friend and associate of Martin Luther King Jr. and agreed wholeheartedly with his policy of direct nonviolent action, with his labelling of racism as a "disease" whose cure could only be nonviolence.[40] And in all her calls for urgent direct action, Smith made ample use of illness as metaphor. She conceived of herself as one of the writers hated by rural white southerners for writing honestly about the South, which is "as irrational as hating a doctor for telling you that you are ill."[41]

Lillian Smith had a 13-year fight with breast cancer from 1953 until her death in 1966 and indeed she used this same disease as a metaphor in the 1950s, the decade when the need was most urgent to find a cure for cancer, an illness that had then been found to be so common and so troubling in the United States. Lillian Smith's crusade for the civil rights of blacks in the 1950s coincided with the efforts of Sidney Farber and Mary Lasker, two oncologists who purposely used the word "crusade" in their battle against cancer. In *The Emperor of All Maladies*, Siddhartha Mukherjee describes this crucial juncture in medical science as "a scientific battle imbued with such fanatical intensity that only a religious metaphor could capture its essence." He adds that "they would stop at nothing to drag even a reluctant nation toward it,"[42] which was essentially the same tactic used by civil rights leaders.

In the pathology of cancer Lillian Smith found an adequate metaphor for the values of the culture of segregation of her native South, a culture which she saw as a type of totalitarianism that harms the whole social

---

[40] David Blight states that James Baldwin, during his visit to the South in 1957, "met Coretta King, whom he admired, at a church basement reception, and listened while the revered [Luther King] explained to his parishioners that racism was a 'disease' and nonviolence its cure." See David W. Blight, *American Oracle: The Civil War in the Civil Rights Era* (Cambridge, Mass.: Harvard University Pres, 2011), 216.

[41] Lillian Smith, *Killers of the Dream*, 192.

[42] Siddhartha Mukherjee, *The Emperor of All Maladies: A Biography of Cancer* (London: Fourth Estate, 2011), 115.

body if it is left unchecked and out of control. In *Illness as Metaphor* (1978) Susan Sontag posits that "it is diseases thought to be multi-determined (that is, mysterious [like cancer]) that have the widest possibilities as metaphors for what is felt to be socially or morally wrong."[43] In the final chapter, originally titled "Disease as political metaphor,"[44] Sontag notes: "Illnesses have always been used as metaphors to enliven charges that a society was corrupt or unjust. Traditional disease metaphors are principally a way of being vehement."[45] Lillian Smith was the most vehement white southern liberal of her time, to the point that she sometimes seemed like the bad psychiatrist who shouts at her "patients." As Sontag says, "The cancer metaphor seems hard to resist for those who wish to register indignation."[46] Cancer is an expansionist disease, like racism or colonialism, which Lillian Smith saw as parallels and described as two cancers that metastasized throughout the world.

In order to avoid metastasis, the expansion of her breast cancer, Lillian Smith bravely and resolutely underwent a radical mastectomy in 1953. She equally saw racism as a malignant growth which would metastasize rapidly and implacably unless radical measures were taken to prevent the total destruction of the whole social body. Consequently, she never had patience with those southerners who demanded slow integration and insisted on a process without interference from the North. On December 5, 1956, the first anniversary of the bus boycott in Montgomery, Alabama, a speech by Lillian Smith was read to the civil rights workers and the organizers of the Institute on Non-Violence and Social Change. In the speech, titled "The Right Way Is Not a Moderate Way," Smith wrote that "moderation never made a man or a nation great. Moderation never mastered ordeal or met a crisis successfully. Moderation never discovered anything; never invented anything; never dreamed a new dream."[47] She lamented that the "so-called moderates are doing nothing," which means that "they are suffering from temporary moral and psychic paralysis."[48] The speech influenced Martin Luther King, who paid close attention to Smith's arguments and kept a copy of the speech among his papers.

---

[43] Susan Sontag, *Illness as Metaphor and AIDS and Its Metaphors* (London: Penguin Books, 1991), 62.

[44] M. Sabini, "Sontag, Susan. *Illness as Metaphor,*" Book review, *Journal of Analytical Psychology* 24 (1979): 272.

[45] Sontag, *Illness as Metaphor*, 73.

[46] Ibid., 84.

[47] Lillian Smith, "The Right Way Is Not a Moderate Way," *The Winner Names the Age*, 68.

[48] Ibid., 72.

Smith faced the same fierce opposition from gradualist white liberals that Luther King faced from accommodationist black leaders. In *Now Is the Time* (1955) she flatly rejects the statement that "segregation cannot be done away with overnight" as "silly": "A house is not built overnight but it is built, often, in six months."[49] Both Luther King and Lillian Smith rejected the gradualists' argument that the natural flow of time will solve all problems; they had a different sense of time, reflected in King's famous assertion in his "Letter from a Birmingham Jail": "We must use time creatively, in the knowledge that the time is always ripe to do right."[50] For Smith, the gradualists were "men who clung to their white culture as a cripple clings to his crutches."[51] Luther King and Lillian Smith were among the first to recognize the importance and the implications of Gandhi's struggle to make British colonial rule in Asia illegitimate. They agreed on the urgent need for political paths that would function as radical alternatives to the trap of moderation that accommodated unjust social conditions. During the same period there was in the U. S. a clash between two approaches to cancer research: the slow approach of Vannevar Bush which consisted of long-term, basic scientific research, of waiting for fundamental questions about cancer to be solved before launching an all-out attack on the problem, and the urgent war on cancer demanded by Mary Lasker and Sidney Farber, who demanded strong commitment by Congress and the nation as a whole.[52] Mukherjee refers to the confrontation as "a deep intellectual divide that ran through the front lines of oncology: the rift between overmoderated caution and bold experimentation."[53]

In the speech "The Right Way Is Not a Moderate Way," which she could not deliver in person because of a momentary aggravation of her cancer, Lillian Smith compared people who fail to react to stop segregation because they are afraid and who prefer to be tactful, with those "who react in a similar way when they are told they have cancer. They decide to be moderate and do nothing; to rock along and postpone thinking about it. Why? Because they are scared. And, because of their fright, they convince

[49] Lillian Smith, *Now Is the Time* (Jackson: University Press of Mississippi, 2004), 91. *Now Is the Time* is Smith's passionate defence of America's moral obligation to civil rights, intended to capitalize on the momentum provided by the 1954 Supreme Court's *Brown v. Board* ruling which outlawed school segregation.

[50] Martin Luther King, Jr., "Letter from a Birmingham Jail," *The Civil Rights Reader: American Literature from Jim Crow to Reconciliation*, ed. Julie Buckner Armstrong (Athens: University of Georgia Press, 2009), 187.

[51] Lillian Smith, *Killers of the Dream*, 136.

[52] Siddhartha Mukherjee, *The Emperor of All Maladies*, 120-21.

[53] Ibid., 130.

themselves that if they do nothing, if they take a few vitamins, maybe, the cancer will go away."[54] She adds that "neither cancer nor segregation will go away while we close our eyes. Both are dangerous diseases that have to be handled quickly and skillfully because they spread, they metastasize throughout the organism." And, being well aware of the interrelations between the individual physical body and the social body, she notes that "We have also seen sick race relations metastasize throughout our country—and indeed, throughout the whole earth."[55]

Lillian Smith's position on segregation is no different from Sidney Farber's on cancer. According to Mukherjee, Dr. Farber's fame grew in part because of his insistence that cancer "was a total disease—an illness that gripped patients not just physically, by psychically, socially, and emotionally."[56] Both are problems that cannot be walled in, and in both cases there is no time to lose in facing them. Lillian Smith's warning to her fellow southerners, then, could not have been more urgent: "How we deal with this critical situation, how we face up to it, will determine our moral health as individuals, our cultural health as a region, our political health as a nation; and our prestige as a leader of democratic forces throughout the world."[57]

With her writings and speeches Lillian Smith undoubtedly awoke many consciences in the United States and her critical views of her country's racial practices contributed greatly to the growing calls for civil and legal transformation of the cancerous racist order during the 1940s and 1950s. But she always conceived of the battle being fought in the South as a battle for civilization, and she stressed the parallels between racial segregation and colonialism, two cancers that blighted the world. She always explored the social evils and the psychological conflicts derived from racialism in America in terms of their connections to other countries and cultures. She was one of the first to see the transnational dimensions of the cultural and racial practices of her region, and one of the first to characterize the white dominance of the South as a colonial relationship. The failure of most southerners to make a decision and forget "the old dead causes" was for her comparable to "the unreasonable way in which the European powers have clung to colonialism even though they know it is a corpse."[58]

---

[54] Lillian Smith, "The Right Way," 69.
[55] Ibid., 69-70.
[56] Siddhartha Mukherjee, *The Emperor of All Maladies,* 125.
[57] Lillian Smith, "The Right Way," 71.
[58] Smith, *Killlers*, 233.

Works Cited

Avary, Myrta Lockett. *Dixie after the War.* New York: Doubleday, Page & Company, 1906.

Blight, David W. *American Oracle: The Civil War in the Civil Rights Era.* Cambridge, Mass.: Harvard University Press, 2011.

Bradatan, Costica. "Scaling the 'Wall in the Head,'" *New York Times* November 27, 2011. http://opinionator.blogs.nytimes.com/2011/11/27/scaling-the-wall-in-the-head/?nl=todayshe

Cliff, Michelle, ed. *The Winner Names the Age: A Collection of Writings by Lillian Smith.* New York: Norton, 1978.

Clinton, Catherine. *Tara Revisited: Women, War, & the Plantation Legend.* New York: Abbeville Press, 1995.

Fredrickson, George M. *The Black Image in the White Mind: The Debate on Afro-American Character and Destiny, 1817-1914.* New York: Harper Torchbooks, 1971.

Gladney, Margaret Rose. *How Am I to Be Heard? Letters of Lillian Smith.* Chapel Hill: University of North Carolina Press, 1993.

Hoffman, Frederick L. *Race Traits and Tendencies of the American Negro.* New York: The Macmillan Company, 1896.

King, Martin Luther, Jr. "Letter from a Birmingham Jail." In *The Civil Rights Reader: American Literature from Jim Crow to Reconciliation,* edited by Julie Buckner Armstrong, 180-93. Athens: University of Georgia Press, 2009.

Kovel, Joel. *White Racism: A Phychohistory.* 1970. London: Free Association Books, 1988.

Loveland, Anne C. *Lillian Smith: A Southerner Confronting the South.* Baton Rouge: Louisiana State University Press, 1986.

Lumpkin, Katharine Du Pre. *The Making of a Southerner.* 1946. Athens: The University of Georgia Press, 1991.

Morrison, Toni. *Playing in the Dark: Whiteness and the Literary Imagination.* 1992. New York: Vintage, 1993.

Mukherjee, Siddhartha. *The Emperor of All Maladies: A Biography of Cancer.* London: Fourth Estate, 2011.

Sabini, M. "Sontag, Susan. *Illness as Metaphor.*" Book review. *Journal of Analytical Psychology* 24 (1979): 270-72.

Smith, Lillian. "Growing into Freedom." *Common Ground* 4, no. 1 (Autumn 1943): 47-52.

—. "Humans in Bondage." In Cliff, 32-55. Originally published in the February, 15, 1944 issue of *Social Action*, published by the Council for Social Action of the Congregational Christian Churches, New York.

—. *Killers of the Dream.* Revised edition. 1961. New York: Norton, 1994.

—. "The Moral and Political Significance of the Students' Non-Violent Protests." In Cliff, 91-99. Speech given at All Souls Unitarian Church, Washington, D. C., April 21, 1960.

—. *Now Is the Time.* 1955. Jackson: University Press of Mississippi, 2004.

—. "Ten Years from Today." In Cliff, 56-66. Commencement address at Kentucky State College, June 5, 1951.

—. "The Right Way Is Not a Moderate Way." In Cliff, 67-75. Speech sponsored by the Montgomery Improvement Association, read at the Institute on Non-Violence and Social Change, on the first anniversary of the bus boycott, December 5, 1956.

—. "Ten Years from Today." In Cliff. 56-66. Commencement address at Kentucky State College, June 5, 1951.

Sontag, Susan. *Illness as Metaphor and AIDS and Its Metaphors.* London: Penguin Books, 1991.

Stockett, Kathryn. *The Help.* 2009. London: Penguin Books, 2010.

Thorpe, Earl E. *The Old South: A Phychohistory.* Durham, N. C.: Seeman Printery, 1972.

Van Evrie, J. H. *Negroes and Negro "Slavery;" The First, an Inferior Race—The Latter, Its Normal Condition. Introductory Number: Causes of Popular Delusion on the Subject.* Baltimore: John D. Toy, 1853.

—. *Negroes and Negro "Slavery:" The First, an Inferior Race: The Latter Its Normal Condition.* New York: Van Evrie, Horton & Co., 1861.

CHAPTER EIGHT

"DON'T TURN THE LIGHT ON!": TENNESSEE WILLIAMS, ILLNESS AND POPULAR CULTURE

RICHARD HAYES

I

Tennessee Williams's notebooks, letters, and the notorious *Memoirs* linger frequently on the many illnesses Williams suffered—or thought he suffered—through his life. His *Notebooks* often read as a litany of sickness after sickness: "I am suffering. Physically. The same condition. Woke me up. What shall I do?" (17 November 1943); "Some twinges here and there in the abdomen" (4 April 1947); "My belly aches a bit in a dull way" (20 October 1947); "I feel very shaky indeed. Had to use liquor … to get through the evening" (8 June 1954); "Physical symptoms alarming. Have bled from bowels four nights in succession" (February 1957).[1] His *Memoirs* and letters similarly record episode after miserable episode; his account of his own life is punctuated by hospitalizations, physical suffering, and real and sometimes imagined pain.

How seriously are we to take Williams when he makes these complaints? One might be inclined to dismiss Williams's relentless grumbling as that of at least a part-time hypochondriac were it not for the frequency with which illness also appears in his work. From Blanche DuBois in *A Streetcar Named Desire* to, most viscerally, Big Daddy in *Cat on a Hot Tin Roof*, many of the central characters in Williams's plays are, to varying degrees, "sick". There is, one can argue, some elements of continuity in this respect between Williams's life and his work, a

[1] Tennessee Williams, *Notebooks*, ed. Margaret Bradham Thronton (New Haven, CT: Yale University Press, 2006), 411, 463, 641, 701.

conclusion supported by Williams's own declaration in his 1955 essay "Person-to-Person", often reprinted as an introduction to *Cat*, that "those emotions that stir him deeply enough to demand expression" are "nearly all rooted, however changed in their surface, in the particular and sometimes peculiar concerns of the artist himself".[2]

It is highly theoretically problematic, of course—as well as unfashionable—to make too much of links between a writer's art and his life. But the leap between the writer's sickness, in this case, and that of his characters is not very far. It has long been recognized that *The Glass Menagerie*, for instance, as well as many other works, are identifiably autobiographical in content—that play contains many direct traces of Williams's own life, particularly his life with his sister Rose who suffered from mental illness and was, in the end, lobotomized and permanently hospitalized.[3] There is, moreover, an important connection between the tragic Rose and Williams's writing: "I don't think I would have been the poet I am without that anguished familial situation", he said at one point.[4] It is not going too far to suggest that Williams's own illnesses, and indeed the illness particularly of Rose, inform, shape, and maybe even explain the plays.

Or, to take another perspective, there would seem at least to be some merit in treating as continuous William's own declarations about his life and the work he produced for the stage. Elsewhere in "Person-to-Person", Williams recalls seeing a group of girls on a Mississippi sidewalk dressed up in their mothers' clothes, "old raggedy ball gowns and plumed hats and high-heeled slippers". He writes:

> One child was not satisfied with the attention paid her enraptured performance by the others, they were too involved in their own performances to suit her, so she stretched out her skinny arms and threw back her skinny neck and shrieked to the deaf heavens and equally oblivious playmates, "Look at me, look at me, look at me!" … I wonder if she is not, now, a Southern writer.[5]

---

[2] Tennessee Williams, "Person-to-Person," *Where I Live: Selected Essays*, ed. Christine R. Day and Bob Woods (New York: New Directions, 1978), 75.
[3] Spoto recounts an interview with Dakin Williams, Tennessee's brother, who claims that "The events of *The Glass Menagerie* … are a virtually literal rendering of our family life." See Donald Spoto, *The Kindness of Strangers: the Life of Tennessee Williams* (New York: Ballantine Books, 1985), 125.
[4] Spoto, 67. Spoto is quoting from an interview with Williams by Cecil Brown in *Partisan Review*, 45 (1978): 276-305.
[5] Williams, "Person-to-Person," 76.

His accounts of his various illnesses are best understood in this context. Many of Williams's plays, it can be suggested, are a self-drama of a kind; in other words, Williams shares the impulse towards self-dramatization with that little girl in the story. It is no coincidence that Tom in *The Glass Menagerie*—a barely disguised version of Williams himself—addresses directly the audience at the start of the play, and the action that follows becomes a playing out of his own life story. The complaint of "twinges" and pain and illness in Williams's notebooks, letters, and essays are a kind of self-drama deserving attention in the context of the more—and sometimes considerably less— hidden self-drama of the plays. In this way, seemingly ephemeral works (letters, notebooks) stand as curious extensions to the plays—and as such are in themselves deserving of critical scrutiny, less for what they tell us about Williams the man but more as extensions of his creative output.

In other words, illness in Williams's work—including his letters and other seemingly secondary material—needs to be read as metaphor and the functioning of that metaphor is in part a concern of this essay—*contra* Sontag, attempts will be made below to "interpret" the metaphor of illness in Williams. (Sontag's strategy, of course, is "against interpretation", her polemic, *Illness as Metaphor*, founded on the notion that the metaphors used to describe illness create a mythology that frustrates rather than enables a cure: "the metaphoric trappings that deform the experience of having cancer … inhibit people from seeking treatment early enough." "The metaphors and myths," she adds, "kill."[6]) More precisely, one form illness takes in Williams's work—some aspects of the form of Blanche DuBois's illness in *A Streetcar Named Desire*—will be examined. While it will be the work of another day to elaborate this examination into a more searching consideration of the illness-related "metaphoric flourishes" (to use Sontag's term[7]) in Williams's work, it is proposed that an examination of the form of Blanche's madness illuminates some new ways of looking at Tennessee Williams's theatre.

II

As in *The Glass Menagerie*, *A Streetcar Named Desire* features Williams's sister Rose in another guise. In some ways, Blanche is a more complete portrait of Rose than Laura is in the earlier play, and in *Memoirs*,

---

[6] Susan Sontag, *"Illness as Metaphor" and "AIDS and its Metaphors"* (New York: Farrar, Strauss and Giroux, 1990), 102.
[7] Sontag, 112.

Williams makes explicit the connection. He recalls walking with Rose in downtown St Louis, drinking root-beer and window shopping: "Rose's passion, as well as Blanche's, was clothes."[8] Blanche hears things, voices, noises, music, gunshots, and displays all the symptoms that Rose seems to have displayed. She lives a kind of half-imagined existence, as did Rose apparently, in which there is a considerable element of sexual fantasy. In one scene in the play, for instance, Blanche seems about to seduce a boy who calls to the door: "Young man, young, young, young, young—man! Has anyone ever told you that you look like a young prince out of the Arabian Nights?… I want to kiss you, just once, softly and sweetly on your mouth…. It would be nice to keep you, but I've got to be good and keep my hands off children."[9] Rose also suffered from what Williams (in Spoto's words) explained as "exclamations of sexual desire deriving from the repression of a sick woman who was almost thirty years old".[10] Spoto goes on to recount an episode where Rose imagined her father had come into her room looking to sleep with her. At the end of *A Streetcar Named Desire*, Blanche is taken away by doctors clearly from a mental hospital, as Rose was; it is not unfair to speculate that a fate like Rose's awaits Blanche.

The interest here lies less in the actual detail of the Rose story, and its accuracy as it manifests itself in Williams's major plays, but in the ways in which the illness manifests itself, particularly in the metaphors used by Blanche in enacting her illness. Of particular interest is Blanche's curious preoccupation with lights as an expression of her mental degeneration. Of course she is trying to hide her age from erstwhile lover Mitch, and avoids the exposure that comes with electric light. But she does so with a level of obsession that is alarming and clearly a product of mental disturbance. "I can't stand a naked light bulb, any more than I can a rude remark or a vulgar action" she says as she has Mitch put a paper shade over the bulb in her room in Scene Three.[11] Later, in Scene Nine, Mitch confronts her about having lied to him. "It's dark in here," he says. "I like it dark. The dark is comforting to me," she replies. He says, "I don't think I've ever seen you in the light…. That's a fact!… Let's turn the lights on in here!", and as he tears the paper lantern down, "*she utters a frightened gasp*."[12]

---

[8] Tennessee Williams, *Memoirs* (London: Allen, 1976), 120.
[9] Tennessee Williams, *"A Streetcar Named Desire" and "The Glass Menagerie,"* ed. E. Martin Brown (Harmondsworth: Penguin, 1959), 70.
[10] Spoto, 66.
[11] Williams, *A Streetcar*, 46.
[12] Ibid., 99.

He wants, he says, to look at her plain; she says, "I don't want realism." "What do you want?", he asks:

> Magic! Yes, yes, magic! I try to give that to people. I misrepresent things to them. I don't tell the truth. I tell what *ought* to be truth. And if that is sinful, then let me be damned for it! – *Don't turn the light on!*[13]

Blanche's obsession with lights must be set within other ways in which dark-light imagery is employed in the play. The darkness is associated in *Streetcar* with sex. Stella recalls Stanley on their wedding night smashing all the light bulbs with a shoe before making love to her—"There are things that happen between a man and a woman in the dark—that sort of make everything else seem—unimportant," says Stella.[14] Blanche wants Mitch sexually; her fear is that if he turns on the light not only will he see her as she really is but the opportunity for intimacy between them will have gone.

Williams makes more explicit this association between darkness and sex in some of his short stories. In "The Mysteries of the Joy Rio" (written in 1941 and the basis of the play *Those are the Stairs You Got to Watch*), a cinema's upper balcony is described as a place of "fun", to be avoided by the innocent where possible. The balcony is a place "where practically every device and fashion of carnality had run riot in a gloom so thick that a chance partner could only be discovered by touch."[15] In "Desire and the Black Masseur", the experience of the movies is similarly depicted in explicitly sexual language. Anthony Burns, the hero of the story, "loved to sit in the back rows of the movies where the darkness absorbed him gently so that he was like a particle of food dissolving in a big hot mouth." Williams's description of the power of the movies is couched in the language of sex: the cinema is like "a big hot mouth" that "licked at his mind with a tender, flickering tongue"; the figures on the screen "warmed him as if they were cuddled right next to him in the dark picture house."[16] In *The Glass Menagerie*, Tom seems to spend all his spare time going to the movies; "*a perfect shower of movie-ticket stubs*" descends from his pocket as he searches for his keys at the beginning of the fourth scene of the play.[17] "Why do you go to the movies so much?" asks his mother; "I

---

[13] Ibid., 100.
[14] Ibid. 58.
[15] Tennessee Williams, "The Mysteries of the Joy Rio," *Collected Stories* (London: Minerva, 1996), 103.
[16] Tennessee Williams, "Desire and the Black Masseur," *Collected Stories*, 205.
[17] Williams, *The Glass Menagerie*, 149.

go to the movies," says Tom, "because—I like adventure."[18] It is clear that the adventure Tom seeks is of a sexual kind.

For Gilbert Debusscher, indeed, the cinema in Williams is associated with "nocturnal impulses so carefully kept under control in the light"—in *The Glass Menagerie*, the cinema ("the place of imagination and freedom where darkness favors temporary togetherness") is contrasted with the warehouse ("a place of regulation and isolation, the epitome of the brightly lit material world of reality").[19] Blanche's plea, "Don't turn the light on!", is a plea for togetherness and imagination and freedom against regulation and loneliness. In other words, the metaphor through which Blanche communicates her illness can be interpreted as a cry against restrictions on imagination. In this sense, it is not unreasonable to read in Blanche's words also a theoretical statement by the playwright, at least a conviction on what art should be about. Certainly this kind of aesthetic informed his approach to *Camino Real*:

> To me the appeal of this work is its unusual degree of freedom. When it began to get under way I felt a new sensation of release, as if I could "ride out" like a tenor sax taking the breaks in a Dixieland combo or a piano in a bop session. You may call it self-indulgence, but I was not doing it merely for myself. I could not have felt a purely private thrill of release unless I had hope of sharing this experience with lots and lots of audiences to come.
>
> My desire was to give these audiences my own sense of something wild and unrestricted that ran like water in the mountains, or clouds changing shape in a gale, or in the continually dissolving and transforming images of a dream.[20]

Blanche's plea for "magic. Yes, yes, magic" could easily be placed then in the mouth of the playwright himself; her "Don't turn the light on!" can be seen as a theoretical, formal statement, a position on style. It recalls, in this, another almost theoretical statement at the start of *The Glass Menagerie* when the narrator, Tom, declares: "Yes, I have tricks in my pocket, I have things up my sleeve. But I am the opposite of a stage magician. He gives you illusion that has the appearance of truth. I give you truth in the pleasant disguise of illusion."[21] Blanche's madness in *Streetcar*

---

[18] Ibid., 154-5.

[19] Gilbert Debusscher, "Tennessee Williams's Dramatic Charade: Secrets and Lies in *The Glass Menagerie*." *Tennessee Williams Annual Review* 3 (2000): 67.

[20] Tennessee Williams, "Foreword to *Camino Real*," *Where I Live*, 64.

[21] Williams, *The Glass Menagerie*, 130.

is then a form of declaration by Williams of the value of fantasy in art and of the importance of resisting realism.

Christopher Bigsby has argued that in their formal experimentation, Williams and Arthur Miller "were concerned to develop a theatrical style which reflected their desire to … trace the social and psychological origins of cultural anxiety"[22] and, very importantly, Williams's most experimental work, *Camino Real*, he introduces as "nothing more nor less than my conception of the time and world that I live in."[23] Bigsby links the kind of formal exhortation issuing from Blanche with larger forces at work in mid-century America. Blanche's plea that the darkness remain, that there not be light, coupled with the association of desire with darkness, suggests a plea for particularly sexual liberation against forces that deny it. Her cry may be a cry from the heart to stay in the dark where passion is possible, where the "magic" of the kind of passion-filled world of sex exists.

Such a plea can be set in the context of post-War American conservatism, where the rise of Joseph McCarthy, for instance, represented to Dwight MacDonald a "melancholy Triumph of Fact".[24] The kind of sexual liberation Tennessee Williams depicts as happening in the back rows of the cinemas of America can be set against what John Cawelti calls the "myth of proper sexuality" which suggested that there was such a thing as proper sex (heterosexual, married, monogamous, domestic), a myth that, by the 1960s, began to be seen to be "giving way to, or at least entering into, some kind of dialectic with a myth of erotic liberation and domination."[25] There is a kind of challenge in Williams to post-World War Two, Cold War American sexual restraint, what Gronbeck-Tedesco identifies as a national strategy where "conformity to sexual constraints became the sign of a country that had girded its loins on behalf of a militant return to normalcy against the Soviet Union and its toxic

---

[22] C. W. E. Bigsby, *A Critical Introduction to Twentieth-century American Drama, 2: Tennessee Williams, Arthur Miller, Edward Albee* (Cambridge: Cambridge University Press, 1984), 7.

[23] Williams, "Foreword to *Camino Real*," 63.

[24] Quoted in Richard H. Pells, *The Liberal Mind in a Conservative Age: American Intellectuals in the 1940s and 1950s*, 2nd ed. (Middleton: Wesleyan University Press, 1989), 330.

[25] John Cawelti, "Pornography, Catastrophe, and Vengeance: Shifting Narrative Structures in a Changing American Culture," *The American Self: Myth, Ideology, and Popular Culture*, ed. Sam Girgus (Albuquerque: University of New Mexico, 1981), 188.

ideology".[26] Blanche's plea, from her sickness, is a kind of political plea against those conservative forces.

One is encouraged in this way to think of Tennessee Williams as a radical playwright and the illness of his characters, as well as his own illnesses, as predominantly ironic in intent: it is not Blanche who is really sick but the world around her; and it is Williams's society that is sick, not Williams himself. However, we cannot ignore that there is something panicked, despairing, and distressing about Blanche's plea, and indeed also about Williams's own complaints in his letters and journals. It is impossible to read Blanche's "Don't turn the light on!" positively, as it were a kind of rallying cry; her tragedy resides precisely in her not being able to turn on the light, in not exposing her truth to the world: one cannot live on lies and she is found out and discovers the world to be a lonely place.

Blanche's plea is also a denial of representation, in some way a resistance to representation: what the dark disallows is the sight of sex, and perhaps what it is she resists is the representation of sex. It is telling in this regard that, while associating sex with the darkness, Stanley and Stella also associate sex with light: "I pulled you down off them columns and how you loved it," he tells Stella, remembering when they first were together, "having them colored lights going!"[27] It is hard to claim that Blanche's reticence is simply prudery—after all, she is not shy of trying to seduce the boy who calls to the door, and she flirts shamelessly with any man who crosses her path. Perhaps it is that Blanche recognizes the poverty of the language, including the visual language, that exists around sex. "Don't turn the light on!" in this sense becomes an anguished cry at the inadequacy of representation.

In the play, indeed, the moment when Stanley and Stella make love is elided by a break between the scenes, the break functioning very much like a movie jump-cut: Scene Four opens with "*the debris of the night before*", including Stanley's pajamas, strewn over the floor, and Stella "*serene in the early morning sunlight.*"[28] The scene where Blanche is raped by Stanley, Scene Eleven, is also skipped over, the scene opening with a "*sky of turquoise.*"[29] So, while Williams might be seen to celebrate sex and sexuality, against "the melancholy Triumph of Fact" that was the McCarthy era, he also clearly establishes parameters around what can be

[26] John L. Gronbeck-Tedesco, "On *The Rose Tattoo*," *Tennessee Williams: A Casebook*, ed. Robert F Gross (New York/London: Routledge, 2002), 67.
[27] Williams, *A Streetcar*, 95.
[28] Ibid., 52.
[29] Ibid., 122.

shown. Blanche celebrates fantasy and the redeeming power of (sexual) imagination, but Williams recognizes the boundaries that permit him being entirely "wild and unrestricted ... like water in the mountains". Geoff Dyer, in the same vein, writes the following about Lawrence's *Lady Chatterley's Lover*:

> An irony attaches to Lawrence's attempts to reclaim the honest language of sex. The battle has been unequivocally won—and Lawrence would, no doubt, have been appalled by some of the consequences of a victory which he, more than anyone else, helped bring about. While writing *Lady Chatterley*, Lawrence had warned his English publisher, Martin Secker, that the novel was "very improper"; by 1968, John Cheever was worried that his new novel, *Bullet Park*, was not improper enough, was, in fact, "very, very clean."... For Lawrence sex was always more than just sex; he had enough of the puritan in him to insist that it had to be the expression of some larger connection of men and women with each other and, ideally, with the living cosmos to boot. As literature has become more and more sexually explicit, so this claim has come to seem harder to sustain ... Lawrence's elaborate evocation of love-making has [in this context] come to seem, if not exactly dated, then almost quaint: a tentative groping for linguistic freedom rather than its consummation.[30]

In 1946, while recovering in hospital from an operation, Williams was visited by Frieda Lawrence. Through his life, he was Lawrentian in sensibility (his early one-act play, "I Rise in Flame, Cried the Phoenix" is a fictional account of Lawrence's death), and this sensibility may well be demonstrated by Blanche's "Don't turn the light on!": for Williams, Blanche's sickness certainly was a plea for freedom, but a freedom towards a greater authenticity of relations between people, not something anarchic. Illness remains illness, in other words, despite the kinds of freedom it seems to promise.

III

Tennessee Williams published a very strange essay in the *New York Times* in November 1946, four days before *Streetcar* opened. The essay, "On a Streetcar Named Success", might be read as a guide to how to view his new, about-to-open play. The essay is a reflection on success (it is often published as a kind of afterword to *The Glass Menagerie*, on which is it a reflection, as "The Catastrophe of Success") and begins with

[30] Geoff Dyer, "DH Lawrence, *Lady Chatterly's Lover*," *Working the Room: Essays and Reviews, 1999-2010* (Edinburgh: Canongate, 2011), 140.

Williams lamenting his life, living in a hotel, dining on room service, being celebrated everywhere he goes. He recounts his despair at the attention he is given for *The Glass Menagerie* and, in the end, says he "got sick of hearing people say, 'I loved your play!' that I could not say thank you" but rather "choked on the words and turned rudely away." He goes on:

> This curious condition persisted about three months, till late spring, when I decided to have another eye operation mainly because of the excuse it gave me to withdraw from the world behind a gauze mask.... Well, the gauze mask served a purpose. While I was resting in hospital the friends whom I had neglected or affronted in one way or another began to call on me, and now that I was in pain and darkness, their voices seemed to have changed ... Once more they were sincere and kindly voices with the ring of truth in them.[31]

Illness here becomes a kind of restorative retreat. It is interesting that it is a retreat furthermore into darkness. His retreat into illness is a retreat from a world of privilege, a retreat from what he calls "the Cinderella myth", "our favorite national myth, the cornerstone of the film industry if not of Democracy itself."[32] The retreat to darkness, and—more importantly, at this point—the celebration of "kindly voices" brings Williams close here, again, to the figure of Blanche who too could only be rescued from her personal despair by the "kindness of strangers."[33]

Williams makes repeated connection in his work between illness and writing and, particularly, between illness, writing and aloneness. In *Memoirs*, Williams writes about his early life and one important change, marked, as many of these changes are, by deterioration in his health:

> My first eight years of childhood in Mississippi were the most joyously innocent of my life.... [But] That world, that charmed time, ended with the abrupt transference of the family to St Louis. This move was preceded, for me, by an illness diagnosed by a small Mississippi town doctor as diphtheria with complications. It lasted a year, was nearly fatal, and changed my nature as drastically as it did my physical health. Prior to it, I had been a little boy with a robust, aggressive, almost bullying nature. During the illness, I learned to play, alone, games of my own invention.[34]

---

[31] Tennessee Williams, "On a Streetcar Named Success," *Where I Live*, 18.
[32] Williams, "On a Streetcar Named Success," 15.
[33] Williams, A Streetcar, 121.
[34] Williams, *Memoirs*, 11.

Important in this passage is not just the sense in which illness annotates a key life-change but also that his consciousness radically alters through the ill health: a "robust, aggressive, almost bullying" boy became, during the illness, a boy who learned to play "games of my own invention." Of course this shift in consciousness marks also the birth of the writer; inventing his own games is naturally a very small step from inventing his own universes and populating them with characters. The link between writing and illness appears often in Williams's *Notebooks* and elsewhere. For instance, an early entry in his notebook (March 1936—he was 25, attending Washington University), reads:

> Today I would like to leave off the record—I was sick tonight—attack of the nervous heart in short story class—got worked up over Prof reading my story aloud—Why I don't know—must learn to control my nerves—didn't last long—I took a pill—still it is always very depressing—makes you feel cut off from the world.[35]

This last sentence is important. A sense of being "cut-off" permeates Williams's work—certainly important characters like Blanche DuBois suffer debilitation because of their seeming isolation—and yet this condition is, in Williams's mind, the distinguishing mark of the writer.

In May 1946 Williams took a trip to Taos during which he was sick and which, after multiple visits to multiple doctors in multiple cities on the way, ended with him in hospital having to undergo surgery. He speaks of this event also in *Memoirs*:

> My friend sat in the hospital with me and I made out my last will and testament while the young doctors shaved my groin for surgery. I had nothing to leave but the playscript of *Battle of Angels* and I left it to my friend. He took the will and tore it to pieces.... I was carted to the operating room. As I went under the ether, I had a sensation of death. I went out trying to tear the ether mask off my face and shouting, "I'm dying, I'm dying."... I have never talked much about that experience in the spring of '46. It marked the beginning of about three years in which I thought I was a dying man. I was so convinced that I was dying that, when Bill Liebling told me, in New York, to buy a new suit, I was reluctant to buy one as I didn't think I was going to live long enough to justify its purchase.[36]

---

[35] Williams, *Notebooks*, 11.
[36] Williams, *Memoirs*, 103-4.

In a letter to his parents about the same set of incidents, his joy—his relief—comes from company. He writes:

> I feel a bit weak and shaky now but otherwise pretty good. Have started working again on my plays. Everyone here has been wonderful, I am never alone, my room is full of flowers. Mabel Dodge Luhan, the local social dictator, paid me a call, Frieda and Brett have called nearly every day and my Mexican friend Pancho has served as Secretary and kept me with books and a radio. The people around here are the kindest I have met.[37]

Once again the narrative that emerges here, and in *Memoirs*, has metaphoric power: to be a writer is to be in some way "ill"; to be "ill" is to be alone, and to be a writer is to be alone; the refuge from that aloneness comes in the form of other people, and yet one cannot be with other people and still write.

Under the gauze bandage, it may be contended, Williams struggled with tensions at the heart of democracy and, specifically, at the heart of the relationship between democracy and art. In this context, it is very telling that Williams drew on the cinema as the medium to represent both "the Cinderella myth" and the "adventure" of sex. H. L. Mencken argues that "the democratic creed asserts that the majority are always right, while the feeling within *avant-garde* culture has always been that the majority are nearly always wrong."[38] For modern American dramatists, there was a disturbing tension between their artistic aspirations and their desire to be democratic (and thus uphold an important American value). Their artistic aspirations seemed to lead modern American dramatists towards holding an elitist position, a position these dramatists were not happy to hold: dramatists through the twentieth century looked with envy at the American film industry and what it could achieve in terms of generating an audience.

At the same time, being democratic seemed to lead American dramatists towards the kind of populism these dramatists associated with Hollywood and other expressions of popular culture and caused various difficulties around their sense of themselves as autonomous artists. Hence the strange dynamic in Williams with regard to success: he retreats from "the Cinderella myth", he insists on writing with "an unusual degree of freedom", yet he succumbs, finally, to success, surrenders to staying in

[37] Tennessee Williams, *The Selected Letters of Tennessee Williams: Volume2, 1945-1957*, eds. Albert J. Devlin and Nancy M. Tischler (New York: New Directions, 2005), 50-1.

[38] Quoted in Marcus Cunliffe, "Literature and Society," *American Literature since 1900*, ed. Martin Cunliffe (London: Sphere, 1975), 378.

high-class hotels. If success sickened Williams, so indeed did failure: "What fearful admission do I have to make, that after 'Streetcar' I haven't been able to write anymore except by a terrible wrenching of the brain and nerves? Now worn out"—so he writes in his notebook for August 1953.[39]

Williams and Elia Kazan, his director, famously took very different views of changes that were made to the first production of *Cat on a Hot Tin Roof*, Williams's most spectacular mid-career success after a number of post-*Streetcar* failures. Williams created the impression that Kazan had tampered with the script for commercial reasons; when it came to publishing the play, Williams insisted on printing two final acts, the "Broadway version" and the version he had originally intended. Kazan, on the other hand, asserted that "It was Williams who wanted the commercial success, and he wanted it passionately."[40] Truth may be more on Kazan's than Williams's side, particularly since Williams had written (referring to *Stairs to the Roof*) of his insistence on never releasing a play "till I felt it had sufficient theatricality to make it commercial. Any play that is not 'commercial'—that is, 'good theatre'—is necessarily still-born, isn't it?"[41]

Something of the same impulse is visible also in "Person-to-Person":

> Of course it is not only Southern writers, of lyrical bent, who engage in such histrionics and shout, "Look at me!" Perhaps it is a parable of all artists.... it is well to be aware of that peril, and not to content yourself with a demand for attention, to know that out of your personal lyricism, your sidewalk histrionics, something has to be created that will not only attract observers but participants in the performance.[42]

Williams had already articulated his concerns around this problem of communication in a letter to Eric Bentley (12 July 1948):

> a general appeal is necessary and can and should be made for the sake of reaching more people without any vulgarization. On the other hand, it is easy for vulgarity to creep in, sometimes without the author's cognizance: there are many entrances for that sly actor![43]

Through Blanche, through her illness—indeed *in* her illness—Williams perhaps points to a "sickness" at the heart of democracy that is also a

---

[39] Williams, *Notebooks*, 583.
[40] Elia Kazan, *A Life* (New York: DeCapo Press, 1997), 544.
[41] Williams is quoted in Allean Hale's introduction to Tennessee Williams, *Stairs to the Roof*, ed. Allean Hale (New York: New Directions, 2000), x.
[42] Williams, "Person-to-Person," 76-7.
[43] Williams, *Letters: Volume 2*, 203.

sickness afflicting stylists in the theatre: how to be both alone and companionable at the same time; how to write for oneself and an audience and satisfy both; how to treasure the populace and resist populism.

Works Cited

Bigsby, C. W. E. *A Critical Introduction to Twentieth-Century American Drama, 2: Tennessee Williams, Arthur Miller, Edward Albee.* Cambridge: Cambridge University Press, 1984.

Cawelti, John, "Pornography, Catastrophe, and Vengeance: Shifting Narrative Structures in a Changing American Culture". *The American Self: Myth, Ideology, and Popular Culture*, edited by Sam Girgus, 182-92. Albuquerque: University of New Mexico, 1981.

Cunliffe, Marcus. "Literature and Society". In *American Literature since 1900*, edited by Marcus Cunliffe, 267-93. London: Sphere, 1975.

Debusscher, Gilbert. "Tennessee Williams's Dramatic Charade: Secrets and Lies in *The Glass Menagerie*." *Tennessee Williams Annual Review* 3 (2000): 57-68.

Dyer, Geoff. "DH Lawrence, *Lady Chatterley's Lover*." *Working the Room: Essays and Reviews, 1999-2010.* Edinburgh: Canongate, 2011. 129-42.

Gronbeck-Tedesco, John L. "On *The Rose Tattoo.*" In *Tennessee Williams: A Casebook*, edited by Robert F Gross,63-78. New York/London: Routledge, 2002.

Kazan, Elia. *A Life*. 1988. New York: DeCapo Press, 1997.

Pells, Richard H. *The Liberal Mind in a Conservative Age: American Intellectuals in the 1940s and 1950s*. 2nd ed. Middleton: Wesleyan University Press, 1989.

Sontag, Susan. *Illness as Metaphor and AIDS and its Metaphors*. New York: Farrar, Strauss and Giroux, 1990.

Spoto Donald. *The Kindness of Strangers: The Life of Tennessee Williams*. New York: Ballantine Books, 1985.

Williams, Tennessee. *Memoirs*. London: Allen, 1976.

—. *"A Streetcar Named Desire" and "The Glass Menagerie,"* edited by E. Martin Browne. Harmondsworth: Penguin, 1959.

—. "Desire and the Black Masseur." *Collected Stories*. 205-212.

—. "Foreword to *Camino Real*." *Where I Live: Selected Essays*. 63-7.

—. "On a Streetcar Names Success." *Where I Live: Selected Essays.* 15-22.

—. "Person-to-Person." *Where I Live: Selected Essays.* 75-80.

—. "The Mysteries of the Joy Rio." *Collected Stories*. 99-109.

—. *Collected Stories*. London: Minerva, 1996.

—. *Notebooks*. Edited by Margaret Bradham Thornton. New Haven, CT: Yale University Press, 2006.

—. *Stairs to the Roof*, edited by Allean Hale. New York: New Directions, 2000.

—. *The Selected Letters of Tennessee Williams: Volume 2, 1945-1957*, edited by Albert J. Devlin and Nancy M. Tischler. New York: New Directions, 2005.

—. *Where I Live: Selected Essays*, edited by Christine R. Day and Bob Woods. New York: New Directions, 1978.

CHAPTER NINE

THE LGBTQ MESSAGE IN *TRUE BLOOD* AND CHARLAINE HARRIS'S *SOOKIE STACKHOUSE* NOVELS

VICTORIA AMADOR

In March 2011, GLAAD (Gay and Lesbian Alliance Against Defamation) recognized the HBO television program *True Blood* as Outstanding Drama Series for its representation and incorporation of LGBTQ characters into its plot lines. This series, an adaptation of Charlaine Harris's *Sookie Stackhouse* novels, premiered in 2008 and has from its inception been extremely popular. Its season-four premiere drew 5.4 million viewers, impressive given that HBO is only in about one third of all US homes,[1] and in June 2014, the seventh and final season of the series will begin. With Harris selling more than one million Kindle e-books through Amazon[2] and no end to the popularity of *True Blood* in sight, the realistic, humorous, sympathetic, and erotic approach the program offers toward the LGBTQ community has not hurt its popularity or its revenue generation. Jacob Klein on his website *HBO Watch* noted in February 2012, just before the start of season five, that the series is one of HBO's top three programs, and that when the program goes into syndication, each episode will earn approximately $800,000. This popularity further demonstrates that viewers embrace the erotic complexities of the program.

GLAAD's recognition of *True Blood*'s message of equality signals the increasing acceptance in American television of such characters, obviating

---

[1] Robert Seidman, "Updated: 'True Blood' Season Four Premiere Averages 5.42 Million Viewers," *TV by the Numbers* (28 June 2011), paras. 1, 3.

[2] Graeme Neill, "Charlaine Harris sells 1 m Kindle e-books," *The Book Seller* (12 May 2011), para. 1.

somewhat the "homosexual panic"[3] linked to the 1980s/AIDS/HIV association of blood exchange in the LGBTQ community with death. In 2010, across all US television programs, gay characters represented 3.9% of all TV characters.[4] That visibility continues, and *True Blood*'s adult approach to the romantic and sexual couplings of the community reflects an increasingly egalitarian perception of the community in American culture. In fact, Charlaine Harris's final novel in the Sookie Stackhouse series, *Dead Ever After*, debuted in May 2013 at number one on the *New York Times* list of hardcover U.S. best sellers.[5]

The primary conceit of this vampire drama is the "coming out of the coffin" of vampires worldwide, thanks to a synthetic blood substitute developed by the Japanese. In the series and in the novels, real vampire blood provides powerful healing, strengthening, and heightened sensuality, and as a result, it is highly sought after and controlled. Vampires are trying to mainstream with "normal" citizens, and the travails of a community of humans and the undead in mythical Bon Temps, Louisiana, form the focus of each week's events.

Given the current fascination with vampires in popular culture, *True Blood*'s popularity is understandable. One of the most unique aspects of the series, however, is its incorporation over seven seasons of a number of gay/lesbian/bisexual characters whose sexuality is not the focus of an individual program but rather another part of the rich panoply of characters, action, and atmospheric entertainment.

This paper will examine the evolving presence of LGBTQ characters in the first five series of *True Blood* and within Harris's novels. Particular attention will be paid to the development and expansion of characters featured in the novels in the television series; the political commentaries in the novels and the programs; and the real-life activism of the actors, novelist and series participants concerning the LGBTQ agenda, helping to obviate the associations of ill health, both physical and mental, within the community.

Those associations have existed for decades, given the institutional definitions of homosexuality as an illness among many conservative churches and religious organizations, within the US military until the Don't Ask, Don't Tell Repeal Act of 2010, and within the psychiatric community. The American Psychiatric Association had listed homosexuality

---

[3] Ellis Hanson, "Undead," Diana Fuss, ed. *Inside/Out: Lesbian Theories, Gay Theories* (London: Routledge, 1991), 324.

[4] James Hibberd, "GLAAD: 'True Blood' has most gay characters," *The Hollywood Reporter* (28 September 2010), para. 4.

[5] "Dead Ever After debuts at top of U.S. best-sellers list," *Reuters* (16 May 2013).

as a mental illness in its official diagnostic manual, The Diagnostic and Statistical Manual of Mental Disorders, Second Edition (DSM II), until 1973, when that diagnosis was removed. "The action was taken following a review of the scientific literature and consultation with experts in the field. The experts found that homosexuality does not meet the criteria to be considered a mental illness,"[6] although changes in cultural perceptions of the LGBTQ community as well as activist protests helped facilitate that turnaround in expert opinion. The view of homosexuality as a mental illness even today among conservatives, combined with the tragedy of HIV/AIDS infections becoming public knowledge in the US in 1981, and with the southern "redneck" stereotyping of "Nancy boys" (Tennessee Williams frequently noted in numerous interviews his father's referral to him as such) makes the "mainstreaming" of the LGBT community in *True Blood* even more remarkable.

Development and Incorporation of LGBTQ Characters

True Blood's egalitarian approach originates in the novels by author Charlaine Harris, whose eleven vampire works (called the *Sookie Stackhouse* novels for their central heroine), created a Louisiana world populated by humans and by vampires "out" both socially and sexually. Harris said in a *New York Times Magazine* interview, "Most of my vampires have experimented with other sexualities....I think that people might be less tense about it if we would all accept the fact that not everyone is wired the same way."[7]

True Blood vividly establishes a contemporary southern Gothic Louisiana landscape in its opening credits sequence, flashing brief images of hot, sultry, daylight swamps, 'gators, and dead possums in the road, and night time images of road houses and illicit couplings.

Light and dark imagery is ubiquitous in both European and Southern Gothic vampire works. The fear of the sun by Harris's creations provides a powerful metaphor of concurrence with the humans seeking shade from the blinding heat of socio-sexual judgment, as well as the cool attraction of the socially-perceived dark side and autonomous identity. The struggle between sunshine and shadow is embodied in Harris's novels and in *True Blood* in the racial and sexual mixes of the central and supporting romantic characters.

---

[6] American Psychiatric Association, "LGBT-Sexual Orientation" (2014), para. 3.

[7] Deborah Solomon, "Once Bitten," *The New York Times Magazine* (30 April 2010), 18.

Their sexual pairings are redolent of traditional European Gothic romances—the blonde heroine—Sookie; the undead hero, Bill the vampire; the pale anti-hero knight—Eric the Viking vampire. At the same time, these characters transform the tropes, reflecting the dis-ease of contemporary society with the Other in all its configurations as well as the disintegration of southern Gothic stereotypes. *True Blood* executive producer Alan Ball, however, has noted that "his vision" is "not…bodice-ripping 'lady porn,' as romance novels are sometimes unfairly branded, but 'about the terrors of intimacy.'"[8]

Sookie initially represents "the ideal southern woman...chaste as [a] cake of ice."[9] Her Caucasian racial profile reflects a traditionally Southern Gothic, hegemonic heroine's profile, yet she is not an aristocratic Creole; she is rather a working-class waitress living with an aging grandmother, whose best friend is the African American, bi-sexual Tara; hence Sookie both reflects and obviates the southern Gothic archetypical heroine as well as Caucasian social dominance. Sookie embodies the new South's contradictions—she is lovely, religious, unsophisticated and dutiful; yet her supernatural gifts—she is telepathic—and quick response to and acceptance of a variety of sexual pleasures offers a contemporary, liberal-minded heroine.

Sookie's ironic, golden-haired innocence provides a visual counterpoint to her first great love, Bill Compton, presented as a predictably brooding brunette, reanimated hero. Just under six feet, he has "thick brown hair...and his long sideburns seemed curiously old fashioned. He was pale, of course; hey, he was dead."[10] Harris's knowing, ironic nod to Byronic expectation provides a humorous reading of light/dark Gothic juxtapositions, and the coupling of Sookie and Bill, as well as Bill's later couplings with various men and women, shatters the boundaries between light and darkness, the living and the undead, and socio-sexual limitations imposed upon minorities.

Eric's blonde beauty further obviates Gothic expectations in that he is "handsome, in fact, radiant; blond and blue-eyed, tall and broad shouldered....Kind of like the guys on the cover of romance books,"[11] although he is much more than the afore-mentioned "lady porn." His looks

---

[8] Dave Itzkoff, "One Sanguine Star," *The New York Times* (16 June 2011), para. 20.

[9] Anne Goodwyn Jones, "The Woman Writer in the South," *The Nineteenth-Century Novel: A Critical Reader*, ed. Stephen Regan (London and New York: The Open University and Routledge, 2001), 481.

[10] Charlaine Harris, *Dead Until Dark* (London: Gollancz, 2004), 2.

[11] Ibid., 119.

align him closely with Sookie, prophesying their later relationship and contradictive personalities. Yet Eric's "maker," the person, who transformed him into a vampire, was a man, and the love they share represents not only the "normalization of the supernatural creature"[12] but also of homosexuality. Eric is actually bisexual (until his amnesiac transformation in *True Blood*'s series four and Harris's *Dead to the World*), dangerously attractive to both genders. That sexual power undermines the purity of the blonde, white male, therefore, while at the same time providing an antagonist who embodies human complexity.

True Blood offers other supporting characters, however, who are Caucasian, African American, and Hispanic American, and their LGBTQ sexuality provides viewers with new templates for engrossing, sympathetic, identifiable characters.

The character of Lafayette, played by Nelsan Ellis, is one of the most fascinating and complex in *True Blood.* With the role expanded from the first novel (where Lafayette is murdered), he is an African American, brazen gay queen who understands and manipulates his cachet as a sexual object, as well being as a loyal employee, friend, and cousin to Tara, who in the original novels is also Sookie's best friend but Caucasian.

Producer Alan Ball decided to expand Lafayette's role because of Ellis's outrageous, creative performance; as he explained, "Nelsan doesn't just improvise, he channels from planet Lafayette. In a lesser actor's hands, Lafayette could come across as extreme or one-dimensional; Nelsan makes him strong, fierce, and deeply lovable."[13] That Lafayette is not a vampire whose homosexuality emphasizes his Otherness, but rather a human being, further helps to present a gay character "who is a more 'truthful' portrayal of homosexuality in the Deep South."[14]

Lafayette also gains a lover in series three and four, a Hispanic American male nurse who also has witch/brujo powers, Jesus Velasquez, played by Kevin Alejandro. Jesus, significantly named, is traditionally masculine yet excels at traditionally feminine roles, their relationship

---

[12] Ewan Kirkland, "Whiteness, Vampires and Humanity in Contemporary Film and Television," *The Modern Vampire and Human Identity*, ed. Deborah Mutch (Houndmills, Basingstoke, Hampshire: Palgrave Macmillan, 2013), 103.

[13] "Inside True Blood," Charlaine Harris, *The Sookie Stackhouse Companion* (London: Gollancz, 2011), 283.

[14] Darren Elliot-Smith, "The Homosexual Vampire as a Metaphor for…the Homosexual Vampire?: *True Blood* Homonormativity and Assimilation," *True Blood: Investigating Vampires and Southern Gothic*, ed. Brigid (Cherry London: I.B. Taurus, 2012), 150.

"progressive in its portrayal of mixed-race, homosexual relations."[15] The puncturing of LGBTQ stereotypes, while featuring people of color, further helps to reinforce healthier perceptions of minorities.

Tara's role also expanded over the first four series. While initially portrayed in the first three series as heterosexual, Tara still had feelings both for Sookie's white brother; for Sam Merlotte, the white owner of the café where she and Sookie work; as well as for Eggs, an African American. After Eggs' death, Tara leaves Bon Temps for New Orleans, and when she returns in Series Four, she is in a lesbian relationship with a fellow cage-fighter and woman of color, Naomi (Vedette Lim). When she becomes a vampire in series five, transformed by the bi-sexual Pam, the manager of the bar Fangtasia, Tara finds a revitalized direction for African American, female power. In the series, Tara sees her mother, a self-absorbed, brutal drunkard, rely on voodoo first and then on an affair with a married black preacher for self-definition. Her cousin Lafayette's unabashedly, delightedly outrageousness is as comforting to her as it is maddening, and their closeness provides wonderful dysfunctional family moments, but his story line takes him to places (like becoming involved with a Hispanic bruja) that make him unavailable to her. Her character appears isolated in the world of Bon Temps, Louisiana, a unique city for its vampire population, but not unusual in its Caucasian supremacy. When she finally gains her fangs, she finds an (eventually) sympathetic maker and her own fiery independence at last, transforming to from victim to victimizer to vamp/ire.

The queen of the Louisiana vampires, Sophie-Anne Leclerq, played by Evan Rachel Wood, is bisexual, and her humor, like Lafayette's, helps create "a complex and ambiguous figure, at once an image of death and an object of desire."[16] She is deeply in love with her female partner, Hadley (Lindsey Haun), who coincidentally is Sookie Stackhouse's cousin, emphasizing the familial blood ties—genetic, vampiric or otherwise--that bind the characters. Sophie-Anne however also approaches Bill as a possible sexual partner, and accomplishes all of this with humor and aplomb. Her character presents a vampire queen somewhat reminiscent of Catherine Deneuve's Yves Saint Laurent-garbed vampire in the 1983 film *The Hunger*; chic meets ruthlessness in both characters.

In Series Three and Four, the Queen is forced through a power struggle to marry the King of the Mississippi vampires, Russell Edgington, who happens to be gay. As played by Denis O'Hare, he is a middle-aged,

---

[15] Ibid., 151.

[16] Andrea Weiss, *Vampires and Violets: Lesbians in the Cinema* (London: Jonathan Cape, 1992), 84.

elegant, ruthless vampire whose husband of 700 years, Talbot (Theo Alexander), is something of a housewife stereotype yet another multi-layered character. While his effeminate fussing about the blood sorbet he serves a dinner guest or his house-proud pleasure in the mansion he shares with Russell mimics a First Lady's wifely duties, Talbot truly loves Russell, and it is mutual. Their quiet moments together are sincere, played for anything but mockery of transgendered roles. Talbot is fierce in his pride and his possessiveness of Russell, no southern belle. Their relationship, Talbot's murder, and Edgington's insane grief has authentic poignancy, thereby investing human depth into the variety of configurations of LGBTQ relationships.

Socio-sexual-political Commentary

The central protagonists are all Caucasian/Anglo/White, and while this clearly reflects the European Gothic tradition, it also reflects traditional Southern power constructs. Harris is Caucasian; Sookie, Harris's first-person narrator, is White. With Harris, one hesitates to presume author-identification with her heroine, but her heroine's race allows Harris to explore the vampire genre and Southern Gothic expectations, as well as approach the social milieu of small-town northern Louisiana, through her own Caucasian perspective.

The horror genre may often feature "white people chomping away at white people,"[17] but Harris and the *True Blood* producers make efforts to broaden not only the feeding habits of their protagonists/vampires, but also to broaden their critique of the Louisiana racial landscape. Just as Hughes notes that Poppy Z. Brite's *Lost Souls* "resolutely refuses to allow vampirism *as* vampirism to function as the central issue of its exploration into the troubled nature of identity,"[18] so too does Harris explore issues of identity within the vampire genre, allowing race and sexuality to function as *a* central issue but not *the* central issue.

The sexuality in Harris's novels reflects the "mutability of erotic experience"[19] which appeared in English vampire literature as early as Samuel Taylor Coleridge's *Christabel* (1816) with its heroine attracted by her male lover as well as the title feminine figure. That mutability

[17] Richard Dyer, *White: Essays on Race and Culture* (London and New York: Routledge, 1997), 211.
[18] William Hughes, "'The taste of blood meant the end of aloneness': Vampires and Gay Men in Poppy Z. Brite's *Lost Souls*," *Queering the Gothic*, eds. William Hughes and Andrew Smith (Manchester: Manchester University Press, 2009), 150.
[19] Joan Acocella, "In the Blood," *The New Yorker* (16 March 2009), para. 19.

continues in the lesbian relationships of Sheridan Le Fanu's *Carmilla* (1872), flows through the blood exchanges of Bram Stoker's *Dracula* (1897), and is transfused into Harris's novels. Thus Harris not only reconfigures the "unchanging quality in Southern heroines [which] is the ideal of chastity"[20] into something more contemporary and realistic but no less enchanting. The intermingling of blood within Harris's works and in *True Blood* demonstrates a transformation of sexuality, as well as race and gender expectations, in twenty-first century America.

Harris acknowledges in her first Sookie Stackhouse novel the influence of Anne Rice's *Interview with the Vampire.* The novel appeared at a significant time in American gay rights—in 1976, when disco flooded the airwaves and social experimentation was flourishing in the first decade after the Stonewall riots of June 1969, when gay patrons of New York City's Stonewall Inn reacted angrily against yet another police raid, resulting in several days of protests, seen then and now as the inspiration for the gay liberation movement. Rice has said, "The year *Interview with the Vampire* was published, a young man…told me he thought [it] was 'the longest sustained gay allegory in the English language.' I was kind of amazed and honoured."[21] Her sensual if not overtly sexual protagonist Louis is created by another man, Lestat, and "interviewed by a boy (presumably in late adolescence) with a tape-recorder. This narrative strategy emphasizes disclosure.... the vampire comes out of the closet."[22]

This approach could be seen to be eerily prescient, given that Lestat's fictional rebirth in 1985 in *The Vampire Lestat* was published at the height of AIDS pandemic; in response, Rice created an even more obviously homosexual hero. Rice's son Christopher is gay, so just as the immortal child in *Interview,* Claudia, embodied Rice's daughter who died young, Lestat provided a template for her son as well as an anti-hero whose proud homosexuality contradicted the homophobic paranoia of his time.

Harris has continued such liberal acceptance of sexual configurations within her fiction. She noted in an interview with Deborah Solomon for the *New York Times*, "Most of my vampires have experimented with other sexualities. Eric, Sookie's lover, was turned into a vampire by a male

---

[20] Marie Fletcher, "The Southern Woman in the Fiction of Kate Chopin," *Louisiana History: The Journal of the Louisiana Historical Association* 7.2 (Spring 1966): 131.

[21] Marlow Stern, "Anne Rice on Sparkly Vampires, 'Twilight,' 'True Blood,' and Werewolves," *The Daily Beast* (23 November 2011), para. 9.

[22] Ken Gelder, "Vampires in the (Old) New World: Anne Rice's Vampire Chronicles," *Reading the Vampire*, ed. Ken Gelder (New York: Routledge, 1994), 109.

vampire who had a sexual relationship with him for many years. Pam [created by Eric] is bisexual. Lafayette is gay."[23] In answer to a question posed by Solomon as to how she, "a married woman with three children who lives in small-town Arkansas... [got] so interested in bisexual vampires," she responded, "Gay rights is just one of the social issues I'm interested in."[24] Humorously, when asked if she is bisexual, Harris replied, "No. I'm sorry. I'm just not that interesting."[25] Her openness demonstrates how

> [i]n the late twentieth and early twenty-first centuries, contemporary women writers of lesbian and queer [and heterosexual] Gothic have engaged directly with ways in which horror figures and boundary breakers can be portrayed and read in ways which further debate about lesbianism and conventional representations of sexuality.[26]

True Blood also allows for consanguinity between races and classes which would have been forbidden by miscegenation laws and social class limitations well into the 20th century in some southern states. Blood and purity have been central to southern American culture for centuries, so the exchange of fluid as well as the healing and sexual powers of vampire blood among the races and sexual preferences represents a new envisioning of the tragic "one drop" blood ideology of the past; the idea of "true blood" can be perceived beyond the synthetic drink of choice of vampires as a concept embracing authentic identities and relationships. "V," the nickname for vampire blood (mirroring club drug Ecstasy, known as "E"), provides sexual excitement for gays and straights, blacks and whites alike, and visitors to the vampire club Fangtasia can find any kind of coupling and penetration they desire without guilt.

The series portrays a society in which blacks and whites, gays and straights, have found a comfortable co-existence, and while this may suggest an idealized, utopian American multiracial perspective,[27] such suggestions within the media can be argued to further the realization of this idealization as well as represent those southern communities which have indeed moved beyond race and sexuality as a primary determiner of personal/interpersonal boundaries. The vampire metaphor here functions

---

[23] Deborah Solomon, "Once Bitten," 18.
[24] Ibid.
[25] Ibid.
[26] Gina Wisker, "Devouring Desires: Lesbian Gothic Horror," Hughes and Smith, 126.
[27] Nicole Rabin, "True Blood: The Vampire as a Multiracial Critique on Post-Race Ideology," *Journal of Dracula Studies* 12 (2010): 71.

as a trope for the destruction of Caucasian and heterosexual hegemony, for integration of minority populations, and for the destruction of racial as well as social/sexual/class purity mythology.

Real Life Activism

Providing additional texture to the series, two of its leading actresses, Anna Paquin and Evan Rachel Wood, came out as bisexual in 2010. Paquin is married to co-star Stephen Moyer and came out as part of the "It Gets Better" campaign after a series of tragic suicides by young gay American teenagers. Wood married actor Jamie Bell; hence these actresses' private lives offer an authentic counterpoint to their fictional characters, refusing to be limited by societal expectations of heteronormativity.

The series' creator, Alan Ball, is an open homosexual who has appropriated the discriminatory, marginalizing experiences of the LGBTQ community as a metaphor for the treatment of the vampires in *True Blood.* The opening credit sequence, for example, features a shot of a cheap roadside sign proclaiming "God Hates Fangs." This is a re-appropriation of the prejudices of the notorious Westboro Baptist Church of Kansas, whose "God hates fags" signage reflects their right-wing, fanatical agenda.

Additionally, in a rather charmingly southern way, Ball has written with Gianna Sobol and Karen Sommer Shalett a cookbook—*True Blood: Eats, Drinks, and Bites from Bon Temps.* This might be considered a rather stereotypically "gay" book to write, but it also reinforces the hospitality and community feeling of an American region which is also known for its warmth and family feeling. As Ball writes, "I grew up in a small town in the South [….] So when I sat down to write a show about the people of Bon Temps, Louisiana, it was no wonder that so much of their lives would revolve around food. It feels tremendously organic for the drama…to go down over…blood cocktails over at Fangtasia."[28] Recipes like the "Bon Temps Bloody Mary" and "Blood Royale" appear to be a direct challenge to homophobia and fear of blood exchange.

The issue of AIDS is not directly addressed in *True Blood*, but a disease called Sino-AIDS is featured in the first series and in Harris's novels; "a variant of the blood-borne immune system disease, it is one of the few illnesses that can affect vampires, leaving them very weak for a

---

[28] Gianna Sobol, et al., *True Blood: Eats, Drinks and Bites from Bon Temps* (San Francisco: Chronicle Books, 2012), 16.

month after drinking the infected blood."[29] The fact that the vampires do not die but do become ill for a while reflects the progress in various contemporary AIDS treatments. In series one, the human lover of one of a group of vampires is infected with Sino-AIDS and allows himself to be bitten by vampires in order to infect them, as revenge for their killing his former lover. His knowing infection of others reflects some sexual improprieties in homo- and heterosexual culture; yet the healing power of unpolluted V, vampire blood, repudiates the negative associations linked with blood within the LGBTQ community.

In addition to Ball and his writers developing the gay, lesbian and bisexual characters in the weekly series (Lafayette, Tara, Queen Sophie, and others) beyond the plotlines of Harris's novels, they have emphasized also the importance of the action "set against a hot, sweaty and beautifully rendered backdrop of a southern, gothic small town."[30] Ball noted, "'I grew up in a semi-small town in the South, and the descriptions of the characters, the way they behaved and spoke, it all felt like something I recognized.'"[31] This was "'another reason I found these stories attractive... They look at that small-town small-mindedness...[and] the way in which certain minorities are demonized and oppressed for political or social gain.'"[32] Thus Ball's adaptation of Harris's novels affirms the power of "Gothic television...in which fear is the sustaining emotion, translated to the viewer through...a certain 'mood' (melancholy, dread, the uncanny), and through an emphasis on impressionist renditions of (troubled) subjectivities."[33] The troubled subjectivities of many mainstream Americans towards the LGBTQ community are challenged weekly in an entertaining yet instructive way by the *True Blood* cast and crew.

Conclusion

The United States continues to move closer toward marriage equality for the LGBTQ community; as of January 2014, seventeen states have legalized same-sex marriage. Additionally, there is an increasingly accepted presence in mainstream entertainment and media of such figures as talk

---

[29] Victoria Koski, "A Guide to the World of Sookie Stackhouse," Harris (2011), 430-31.
[30] Shelagh Delaney, "The Blood, the Bad and the Ugly," *The Guardian* (11-17 July 2009), 8.
[31] "Inside True Blood," 283.
[32] Delaney 8.
[33] Helen Wheatley, *Gothic Television* (Manchester: Manchester University Press, 2006), 163.

show host Ellen DeGeneres and television comedian Neil Patrick Harris (who portrays a straight lothario in *How I Met Your* Mother); DeGeneres is hosting the ultimate in show business establishment festivities—the Oscars broadcast—for the second time in March 2014. Neil Patrick Harris has hosted the televised Tony awards four times with tremendous success (he has won three Emmys for his efforts), including dancing and singing in an opening production number at the 2011 awards about theatre entitled "It's Not Just for Gays Anymore." Oscar winner Jodie Foster (whose public acknowledgment of her lesbianism has been subtle), actress Maria Bello (her decision to come out in a *New York Times* essay was because her son "asked [her] if there was something [she] wasn't telling him,"[34] *Juno* star Ellen Page, and film and Broadway actor Zachary Quinto are all out and all working. There is even a new television program about two gay fathers and their surrogate mother entitled *The New Normal*, as well as the continuing popularity of *Modern Family* and its gay family.

Yet the movement toward parity in all roles of American life has a long way to go. During the 2012 Republican candidacy race for the presidency, right-wing religious conservative Rick Santorum compared gay relationships to bestiality, declaring, "'You know, man on child, man on dog, or whatever the case may be,'" as well as affirming, "'Diversity creates conflict. If we celebrate diversity, we create conflict.'"[35] In May 2013, the Texas state senate passed "a bill that advocates say unfairly targets transgender people by restricting the forms of identification that can be used to apply for a marriage license in the state."[36]

Hence television programs like *True Blood* embody significance beyond mere entertainment, wherein the "potentially uncomfortable truths about persistent Southern racism and homophobia can be safely discussed within *True Blood*'s fantasy context."[37] *True Blood* fearlessly presents the humanity of its LGBTQ mortal and immortal characters in all of their beauty and vulnerability, flaws and failings. That the program regularly draws over five million viewers per episode and the first season of the program earned over $26 million dollars when released on DVD (Klein) indicates that a wide demographic enjoys the program and has no issues

---

[34] Maria Bello, "Coming Out as a Modern Family," *The New York Times* (29 November 2013), para. 1.
[35] Richard Schiffman, "The Goofiest Things That Rick Santorum Has Said So Far," *The Huffington Post* (27 Feb. 2012), paras. 17, 21.
[36] Sunnivie Brydum, "Transphobic, Antigay Bills Creep into Texas Senate," *The Advocate* (15 May 2013).
[37] Mikel J. Koven, "'I'm a Fairy? How Fucking Lame!': *True Blood* as Fairytale," Cherry 65.

with the LGBTQ sexuality (not to mention heterosexuality) and community issues portrayed. The microcosmic world the characters inhabit signifies the wider world of all of us.

As written in the Bible, and as Dracula reiterated in Bram Stoker's eponymous novel, "The blood is the life."[38] The same blood flows through all of our veins, whatever our race, ethnicity, religious orientation, or sexual preference may be, and in their very important way, *True Blood* and Charlaine Harris's novels reiterate that sexually, socially and spiritually healthy message.

Works Cited

Acocella, Joan. "In the Blood." *The New Yorker*, March 16, 2009. Accessed February 12, 2012. http://www.newyorker.com/magazine/2009/03/16/in-the-blood

American Psychiatric Association. "LGBT-Sexual Orientation." 2014. Accessed February 15, 2014. http://www.psychiatry.org/lgbt-sexual-orientation

Bello, Maria. "Coming Out as a Modern Family." *The New York Times*. 29 November 2013. Accessed February 15, 2014. http://www.nytimes.com/2013/12/01/fashion/coming-out-as-a-modern-family-modern-love.html

Brydum, Sunnivie. "Transphobic, Antigay Bills Creep into Texas Senate." *The Advocate*, May 15, 2013. Accessed May 15, 2013. http://www.advocate.com/politics/2013/05/15/transphobic-antigay-bills-creep-texas-senate

Cherry, Brigid. *True Blood: Investigating Vampires and Southern Gothic.* London: I. B. Taurus, 2012.

"Dead Ever After debuts at top of U.S. best-sellers list." *Reuters,* May 16, 2013.

Delaney, Shelagh. "The Blood, the Bad and the Ugly." *The Guardian*, July 11-17, 2009, 6-8.

Dyer, Richard. *White: Essays on Race and Culture.* London and New York: Routledge, 1997.

Elliot-Smith, Darren. "The Homosexual Vampire as a Metaphor for… the Homosexual Vampire?: *True Blood*, Homonormativity and Assimilation." Cherry, 139-54.

[38] King James Version.

Fletcher, Marie. The Southern Woman in the Fiction of Kate Chopin. *Louisiana History: The Journal of the Louisiana Historical Association* 7.2 (Spring 1966): 117-132.

Fuss, Diana, ed. *Inside/Out: Lesbian Theories, Gay Theories*. London: Routledge, 1991.

Gelder, Ken, ed. *Reading the Vampire*. London and New York: Routledge, 1994.

—. "Vampires in the (Old) New World: Anne Rice's Vampire Chronicles." Gelder, 108-23.

GLAAD Media Awards. March 19, 2011. Accessed February 12, 2012. http://www.glaad.org/mediaawards/22/ny

Hanson, Ellis. "Undead." Fuss, 324-40.

Harris, Charlaine. *Dead until Dark*. London: Gollancz, 2004.

—. *The Sookie Stackhouse Companion*. London: Gollancz, 2011.

Hibberd, James. "GLAAD: 'True Blood' Has Most Gay Characters." *The Hollywood Reporter*. 28 September 2010. Accessed January 4, 2012. http://www.hollywoodreporter.com/news/glaad-true-blood-has-most-28497

Hughes, William and Andrew Smith, eds. *Queering the Gothic*. Manchester: Manchester University Press, 2009.

Hughes, William. "'The taste of blood meant the end of aloneness': Vampires and Gay Men in Poppy Z. Brite's *Lost Souls*." Hughes and Smith 150-9.

"Inside True Blood." Harris, *The Sookie Stackhouse Companion*, 281-8.

Itzkoff, Dave. "One Sanguine Star." *The New York Times*, June 16, 2011. Accessed January 4, 2012. http://www.nytimes.com/2011/06/19/arts/television/anna-paquin-true-blood-star-grows-up.html

Jones, Anne Goodwyn. "The Woman Writer in the South." Regan, 2001 [1981], 481-4.

Kirkland, Ewan. "Whiteness, Vampires and Humanity in Contemporary Film and Television." Mutch, 93-110.

Klein, Jacob. "Why *True Blood* Won't Be Canceled Any Time Soon." *HBO Watch*. 21 Feb. 2012. Accessed April 14, 2013. http://hbowatch.com/why-true-blood-wont-be-canceled-any-time-soon/

Koski, Victoria. "A Guide to the World of Sookie Stackhouse." Harris, 313-461.

Koven, Mikel J. "'I'm a Fairy? How Fucking Lame!': *True Blood* as Fairytale." Cherry, 59-73.

Mutch, Deborah. *The Modern Vampire and Human Identity*. Houndmills, Basingstoke, Hampshire: Palgrave Macmillan, 2013.

Neill, Graeme. "Charlaine Harris Sells 1m Kindle e-books." *The Book Seller.* May 12, 2011. Accessed April 1, 2013. http://www.thebookseller.com/news/charlaine-harris-sells-1m-kindle-e-books.html

Rabin, Nicole. "True Blood: The Vampire as a Multiracial Critique on Post-Race Ideology." *Journal of Dracula Studies* 12 (2010): 63-81.

Regan, Stephen, ed. *The Nineteenth-Century Novel: A Critical Reader.* London and New York: The Open University and Routledge, 2001.

Schiffman, Richard. "The Goofiest Things That Rick Santorum Has Said So Far." *The Huffington Post.* February 27, 2012. Accessed March 14, 2012.http://www.huffingtonpost.com/richard-schiffman/rick-santorum-statements_b_1293657.html

Seidman, Robert. "Updated: 'True Blood' Season Four Premiere Averages 5.42 Million Viewers." *TV by the Numbers*, June 28, 2011. Accessed January 10, 2012. http://tvbythenumbers.zap2it.com/2011/06/28/true-blood-season-four-premiere-averages-5-42-million-viewers/96730/

Sobol, Gianna, et al. *True Blood: Eats, Drinks and Bites from Bon Temps.* San Francisco: Chronicle Books, 2012.

Solomon, Deborah. "Once Bitten." *The New York Times Magazine*, April 30, 2010, 18.

Stern, Marlow. "Anne Rice on Sparkly Vampires, 'Twilight,' 'True Blood,' and Werewolves." *The Daily Beast*, November 23, 2011. Accessed January 7, 2012. http://www.thedailybeast.com/articles/2011/11/23/anne-rice-on-sparkly-vampires-twilight-true-blood-and-werewolves.html

Wheatley, Helen. *Gothic Television.* Manchester: Manchester University Press, 2006.

Weiss, Andrea. *Vampires and Violets*: *Lesbians in the Cinema.* London: Jonathan Cape, 1992.

Wisker, Gina. "Devouring Desires: Lesbian Gothic Horror." Hughes and Smith, 120-31.

CONTRIBUTORS

Victoria Amador earned her doctorate in creative writing and American literature from the University of Denver. She is an Assistant Professor of English at the American University of Sharjah. Her research interests include feminist discourses in classical Hollywood cinema, vampire and Gothic representations in British and American film and literature, and fashion history. She has held two Fulbright senior lectureships in American literature, received three teaching awards, and has worked as a professor as well as administrator in international higher education for over thirty years. Amador is also one of the co-editors of *SXSE* Magazine, an online publication on photography of the American South, and a long-time member of the National Book Critics Circle. Currently she is writing a critical biography of the actress Olivia de Havilland for the University of Kentucky Press.

Marcel Arbeit is Professor in the Department of English and American Studies, Palacký University, Olomouc, Czech Republic. His main fields of research are contemporary southern literature and Canadian cinema. He is the author of a monograph on the novels of Fred Chappell and Cormac McCarthy published in 2006 (in Czech) and the main editor of the three-volume *Bibliography of American Literature in Czech Translation* (2000). His recent publications focus on Doris Betts, Fred Chappell, Harry Crews, Richard Ford, Lewis Nordan, Flannery O'Connor, Chris Offutt, and Elizabeth Spencer; he co-edited *The Mississippi Quarterly* special issue on Lewis Nordan (2007, with Thomas Ærvold Bjerre) and *The (Un)Popular South* (2011, with M. Thomas Inge). Between 2005 and 2013 he was the President of the Czech and Slovak Association for American Studies. He translated into Czech, among other things, Flannery O'Connor's *Wise Blood*, Lewis Nordan's *Music of the Swamp* and *Wolf Whistle* and a selection of Fred Chappell's stories for a volume he also edited.

Thomas Ærvold Bjerre is associate professor in American Studies at the University of Southern Denmark. His research focuses on American popular culture with a particular interest in the American South, the Western, and representations of 9/11 and the War on Terror in popular culture. He has published on southern literature and film in *Mississippi*

Quarterly, *The Appalachian Journal*, and *American Studies in Scandinavia* and has contributed to *Still in Print: The Southern Novel Today*, *Perspectives on Barry Hannah, Larry Brown and the Blue Collar South* as well as the forthcoming *The Rough South: Artistic Representations* and *The South in Fiction and Film: Essays in Adaptation.*

Susanna Delfino is former professor of American history at the University of Genoa, Italy, with which she continues to be affiliated as member of the Faculty Board for the Doctoral Program in Political Sciences. She also collaborates with the University of Florence in advanced teaching activities on U.S. history. A specialist in the economic and social history of the antebellum South, Delfino is the author of four monographs published in Italy and of several articles in the United States, some of which are included with collections of essays. She co-edited *Neither Slave nor Free: Working Women of the Old South* (2002), and three volumes of the series "New Directions in the History of Southern Economy and Society": *Global Perspectives on Industrial Transformation in the American South* (2005), *Technology, Innovation, and Southern Industrialization* (2008), and *Southern Society and its Transformations, 1790-1860* (2011).

Jan Nordby Gretlund is Associate Professor at the Centers for American and English Studies, University of Southern Denmark. He is the author of *Eudora Welty's Aesthetics of Place* and of *Frames of Southern Mind: Reflections on the Stoic, Bi-Racial & Existential South* (essays). He has co-edited five books: *Realist of Distances: Flannery O'Connor Revisited; Walker Percy: Novelist and Philosopher; Southern Landscapes; The Late Novels of Eudora Welty;* and *Flannery O'Connor's Radical Reality*; and he has edited *Madison Jones' Garden of Innocence; The Southern State of Mind*; *Still in Print: The Southern Novel Today*, and two special 'Southern Issues' of *American Studies in Scandinavia.* A collection of his new essays, *Heads on Fire*: *Essays on Southern Fiction*, will be in print in the fall of 2014.

Constante González Groba is Professor of American literature at the University of Santiago de Compostela (Spain). He is the author of a book on the novels of Carson McCullers, in Spanish, and has written essays and book chapters on Herman Melville, Carson McCullers, Stephen Crane, Lee Smith, Lillian Smith, Elizabeth Madox Roberts, Bobbie Ann Mason, Ellen Glasgow and others. His latest book is *On Their Own Premises: Southern Women Writers and the Homeplace* (Universitat de Valéncia,

2008). He edited the book *Hijas del Viejo Sur: La mujer en la literatura del Sur de los Estados Unidos* (Universitat de Valéncia, 2012), to which he contributed an introduction and two chapters, as well as *Unsteadily Marching On: The US South in Motion* (Universitat de Valéncia, 2013), a collection of essays by American and European southernists.

Richard Hayes is Head of the School of Humanities at Waterford Institute of Technology, Ireland, where he also lectures in English literature and Theatre Studies. He has published widely on American theatre and cinema and has a particular interest in the work both of Eugene O'Neill and Tennessee Williams. He also has research interests in contemporary Irish writing, particularly contemporary Irish theatre, and in popular culture and its reception. He is a lead member on a number of Ireland-US research initiatives and currently he heads a research project at WIT investigating the relationship between regional identity and performance.

Renata Nowaczewska is Assistant Professor of History and American Studies at Szczecin University, Poland. She has published articles, book chapters on philanthropy in an international context, social welfare, foundations and their interactions with the government/-s. Her award-winning book on public and private unemployment relief during the Great Depression discusses the role private foundations and community funds played in cooperation with/ opposition to H. Hoover's and F. D. Roosevelt's relief efforts.

Her interests lie within the history of philanthropy, foreign aid, social history and intellectual history, exchange programs in particular and the role international actors play within broadly defined transnational relations. Her current book project explores the mechanisms of reinforcing/implementing democratic values through the exchange programs and other cultural activities during the Cold War period in countries such as Germany, Austria, Italy, Poland, Czechoslovakia and Hungary. She has explored the role foundations, Ford and Rockefeller Foundations in particular, played in organizing help to the refugees and escapees from the Eastern Europe.

Gérald Préher is Associate Professor at the Institut Catholique de Lille (France) and a member of Jacques Pothier's research center "Suds d'Amériques." He defended a doctoral dissertation entitled "The Timelessness of the Past in Southern Literature as Presented in Works by Walker Percy, Peter Taylor, Shirley Ann Grau and Reynolds Price" (which was published in French), and has written several essays on southern literature and film adaptations. He also co-edited books on southern short stories, on writers such as William Faulkner, John Steinbeck, Ernest J. Gaines, Richard Ford, and on women writers in the South. He is currently working on Elizabeth Spencer, Joan Williams and Lisa Alther.

Beata Zawadka is Associate Professor in the Department of English at Szczecin University, Poland. She earned her Ph.D. from the University of Łódź, Poland. Her doctoral dissertation was on the work of Peter Taylor, particularly the identity of his woman characters. She specializes in southern studies, mass culture/media studies, cinema studies (the theory of film genres), and performance studies. As a zealous Francophile, Beata Zawadka adds French studies to the scope of her ongoing postdoctoral research project. The latter will be entitled *Stage/y Region. The U.S. South as Performance.* She is a member of the IASA, EAAS, PAAS, and of the Southern Studies Forum of the EAAS. Dr. Zawadka has presented at and organized conferences in the European Union and beyond and has also published – in Poland and abroad – on topics linked to her field of interest.

INDEX

Literary works are indexed under the author's name, not the title.